# DISMANTLING
# CANCER

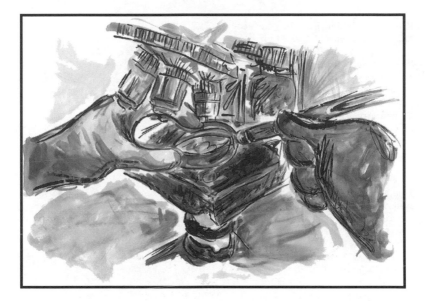

Francisco Contreras, MD,
Jorge Barroso-Aranda, MD, PhD
Daniel E. Kennedy

DISMANTLING CANCER
by Francisco Contreras, MD, Jorge Barroso-Aranda, M.D., Ph.D., and Daniel E. Kennedy
Published by Interpacific Press
1685 Precision Park Lane, Suite L
San Diego, CA 92173
Tel. (800) 950-6505
Tel. (619) 428-0930
Fax. (619) 428-0994


Publisher & Editor: Daniel E. Kennedy
Editorial Coordinator: Luisa Ruiz
Researchers: Jorge Barroso-Aranda, M.D., Ph.D., Jaime Chávez, MT
Writing Staff: Michael Wood and Luisa Ruiz
Graphic Design: Haydeé Aceves Carrillo
Cover Design: Haydeé Aceves Carrillo, Daniel E. Kennedy, Ricardo Álvarez,
Eduardo Gamboa and Laura Monroy Amor
Graphic Art: Haydeé Aceves Carrillo
Photography: Antonio Leyva, www.fotoleyva.com
Format: Laura Monroy Amor

International Standard Book Number: 1-57946-005-4

This book is not intended to provide medical advice or to take the place of medical advice and treatment from your personal physician. Readers are advised to consult their own doctors or other qualified health professionals regarding the treatment of their medical problems. Neither the publisher nor the author takes any responsibility for any possible consequences from any treatment, action or application of medicine, supplement, herb or preparation to any person reading or following information in this book. If readers are taking prescriptions medications, again, they should consult with their physicians and not take themselves off of medicines to start supplementation or nutrition program without the proper supervision of a physician.

Printed in the United States of America

*To Ernesto Contreras Sr., MD*
*(1915-2003)*

*You and your smile, Dad, are greatly missed*
*in the halls of the Oasis of Hope Hospital.*
*Your family, friends, and patients will never forget you.*
*Thank you for leaving a legacy of faith, hope, and love.*
*Your greatest medicine was your unconditional love*
*for your patients.*

# ACKNOWLEDGEMENTS

Since 1994, I have had the opportunity to write ten books. I have been blessed with a wonderful writing team, research team, and design team that have made these publications possible. *Dismantling Cancer* is a book that shares the essence of the forty years of cancer treatment at the Oasis of Hope Hospital that was founded by my father, Dr. Ernesto Contreras, Sr. This book is very special to me because it contains ideas and significant contributions by two of my closest collaborators, Dr. Jorge Barroso-Aranda and Daniel E. Kennedy.

Dr. Barroso-Aranda is the director of my clinical research organization. He is the product of an education at the University of California Berkley, a degree in Engineering from Mexico's top university—the Monterrey Institute of Technology—, a medical degree from UABC, and a Ph.D. in Bioengineering from the University of California San Diego. This gentleman brings a serious scientific background and leadership to all that is done at the Oasis of Hope. It is a privilege to work with him.

Daniel E. Kennedy is the Chief Executive Officer of the Oasis of Hope Health Group and he has been the master builder of my institution since 1993. His background in economics combined with a Master in Business Administration has put Oasis of Hope on a path of continuous improvement. His coursework in ministry and counseling, coupled with his current pursuit of a specialty in psychosocial oncology, is helping me shape what will be the future of the Oasis of Hope integrative cancer treatment approach.

I wish to thank my incredible writer, Michael Wood, who makes our books much more readable, accurate, and interesting. Luisa Ruiz has contributed countless hours to this book and she is just a joy to work with. Thank you Jaime Chávez for the help with research. I am thrilled with the way Haydeé Aceves and Laura Monroy Amor enhance the visual communication of the book. I also thank Ricardo Álvarez, Eduardo Gamboa, María Bernal, and Gloria Rojo for all of their support as well.

# INTRODUCTION

Donald Factor, son of the famous Hollywood make-up artist Max Factor, was diagnosed with cancer in 1986. His doctors told him he would probably not survive. Nothing could have been further from the truth. Donald Factor is alive today, living life to the fullest with his wife Anna. In one of his recent visits to the Oasis of Hope Hospital, he shared his story.

"I was living ninety miles outside of London in November of 1986 when I was diagnosed with carcinoma of the lung that had spread to my liver. The doctors in England didn't hold a lot of hope for me. They were very apologetic and offered a treatment which they thought might extend my life for a little while, but not for very long. I didn't feel like accepting that prognosis and decided to go and see Dr. Contreras. I'd met Dr. Contreras a few years before in a conference my wife and I had helped organize at Warwick University. I was very impressed with his approach. He told us he used modern medicine combined with natural therapies and a lot of love and faith. My wife Anna and I traveled from England to Los Angeles and then we drove down to Tijuana to the hospital where I was treated. When I arrived I was in an extremely weak condition. It was ten days after the original diagnosis and the cancer had spread to my spine. I was in excruciating pain . My sciatic nerve had been affected so I could hardly walk. I was loosing weight rapidly too. They took a look at me at the Contreras clinic and were quite concerned. They were not very optimistic about my future either, but as Dr. Contreras Sr. said, because both I and my wife were very committed to doing everything possible to beat the cancer, they were prepared to work with us. To make a long story short, we succeeded.

I was very impressed with Dr. Contreras' clinic when I went inside and met the people. I had never experienced a hospital where the doctors would treat me as a human being instead of a bunch of symptoms or a disease walking through the door. There was a team of people there who were interested in me and they were involving me in the course my treatment would take. I was being asked, I was being informed and suddenly I was part of the team that was treating me. I wasn't just an object that was being treated. That was tremendous.

Dr. Contreras assured me that the therapy ought to prove helpful immediately. I asked him about laetrile, and he told me that he did not regard it as a silver bullet. It was just one part of his whole metabolic approach to treating cancer. My condition, he told me, was serious and the treatment would be complex. About a week into the course of treatment, which began with a program of detoxification, Dr. Francisco Contreras, his son who is a surgeon and oncologist, performed a minor surgical procedure that involved the insertion of a catheter into my liver to feed laetrile, vitamin C, and a chemotherapy agent directly to the point where they would do the most good. At the time, this was considered a radical new idea. He explained that he only used chemotherapy as a last resort and then only in the minimum amount necessary. His method of treatment was much more precise and also much less aggressive than conventional applications of cancer treatment.

Dr. Contreras also prescribed a week of radiation treatments targeting the tumor on my spine. It was clear that the pain this tumor was causing me was compromising my emotional strength. He explained that the treatment would shrink the tumor, reduce the amount of pain I was dealing with, and strengthen the bones in the process. It did.

I learned later from some of the doctors at the Oasis of Hope that I was more riddled with cancer than any case they had seen before. There were quite a few times during the treatment process when I felt like giving up, and the guilt I felt for even entertaining those thoughts often weighed heavily on me. However, part of the program involved the counsel of a psychologist, who helped me to accept those emotions as a normal part of the healing process. This did much to relieve my guilt and raise my spirits considerably. Dr. Contreras said that my positive and determined attitude along with Anna's enthusiasm helped me immeasurably.

After the initial treatment and about a year of home therapy, I was totally clear of any sign of cancer. Although I will probably never know if any one part of my experience was the actual key to my recovery, I am convinced that it was most likely all of it—everything, physical, emotional and spiritual.

Many orthodox physicians consider metabolic therapy to be out on the fringe. But the theory behind it seems to me like just good common sense. Get the patient well enough to help deal with the disease. Simple. Oncologists seem to have an attitude that ignores the patient and focuses on the disease. Their attitude is, 'If I can't help the patient, nobody can.' Well, I am happy to say that I am living proof that somebody can. For this I will be forever grateful."

**—Donald Factor**

Mr. Factor experienced the eclectic system that integrates conventional, alternative and holistic therapies with the goal of dismantling cancer. The Contreras total care approach has been under development for forty years. This book is an overview of the discoveries, insights and philosophy of a unique comprehensive cancer treatment that has reached its four-decade milestone.

# TABLE OF CONTENTS

Introduction

1. Cancer Mythology ..................................................... 13

2. A Need for Change .................................................. 17

3. The Road Less Traveled ........................................... 27

4. Good Medicine ....................................................... 37

5. Coming Into Focus .................................................. 47

6. Natural Defense System ............................................ 51

7. Cleaning House ....................................................... 57

8. Nature's Pharmacy .................................................. 63

9. A Combined Effort .................................................. 75

10. Something In The Air .............................................. 89

11. Seeing The Light .................................................... 95

12. It's Emotional ........................................................ 101

13. Mind Medicine ...................................................... 105

14. Learning New Tricks ............................................... 113

15. True Spirit ............................................................. 117

16. Great Expectations ................................................. 121

17. Take Charge ............................................................ 129

Epilogue ........................................................................ 131

Appendices ................................................................... 135

References .................................................................... 139

# CHAPTER ONE

## Cancer Mythology

Mythology is an ancient, traditional story or tale about heroes or supernatural beings, often depicting true aspects of life or human behavior that many times are widely believed in but are, in fact, fictitious. Nevertheless, myth plays an important role in the advancement of the sciences and arts. John Maxwell says that "the depth of your mythology is the extent of your effectiveness."[1] I would agree that the many cancer stories researchers have told us have promoted the advancement of knowledge about cancer, but the promised cure is still a myth. Is cancer research history largely an account of mass publications at the expenditure of vast resources to cope with mythical hopes? Well, let me tell you that many of the fears are myths as well.

I do not like to watch television programs, especially sit-coms, but a good movie is something that I cherish, I even will wait in line, something that I truly hate, at the box office or the video store to catch a good one. HBO's mini-series *Band of Brothers* was worth the wait at the counter when the entire collection was released for sale. On the surface, it chronicles the lives of a company of American soldiers during World War II, but the film series is much more. It is an incredible tribute to the ability of the human spirit to overcome tremendous hardship, devastating loss, and seemingly insurmountable opposition. A history of mythic proportions.

I love the story of *Band of Brothers,* not just because I am a World War II buff, or a Steven Spielberg fan. I love the story because I know it so well. I love it because it is the story of every single

13

cancer patient who has walked through the front doors of the Oasis of Hope Hospital where I have spent the bulk of my professional career. I love it because it is the story of every person who has ever battled serious, degenerative disease. But most of all, I love it because it is my father's story.

As a young physician, my father pursued excellence with a tenacity the rival of which I have yet to see. By the 1960s, his reputation had grown to international proportions. He was regarded as one of the most promising young doctors in the field of oncology. Yet, it did not take long for my father to become disenchanted with the poor results yielded by conventional cancer treatment methods. He saw the devastating effect the therapies had on his patients' quality of life, but saw little decrease in the rate of mortality.

Undaunted, my father began to explore the use of alternative therapies to treat cancer. The resistance from his colleagues in the mainstream medical community was intense. In fact, by 1963, he had become a pariah in the field, ostracized completely because he wanted to investigate unconventional treatment methods. This widespread rejection from colleagues was a huge loss to my father, but it did not quench his drive to find and promote treatment methods that alleviated suffering and held more promise than failing conventional therapies. My father battled cancer from the first day of his professional career until the day he died. His story gives me inspiration. It gives me direction. Most of all, it gives me hope.

Recently, I was in Dallas to give an interview on FOX News. I was prepared to answer the standard questions about the potential effectiveness of some of the new treatments on the horizon. I was a little taken aback with the opening question. "What is the biggest myth that still exists about cancer?" the reporter asked, looking me straight in the eyes.

What surprised me the most was not the unexpected nature of the question, but how easy it was to answer. I responded immediately, "The principle myth about cancer is that there is no hope. People feel like they are given a death sentence when they are diagnosed with cancer. They walk around saying, 'I know that you see me here but I am really dead.' But, there are so many things that can be done to either reverse the cancer or significantly improve quality of life for the patient." Like my father before me, I am determined to bring this message of hope to a world that desperately needs it.

It is not hard to understand why most cancer patients adopt a fatalistic view. Both the incidence of cancer and the mortality rates of the disease are daunting. While early detection technologies have definitely made a positive impact, the world continues to wait for a significant breakthrough. Why isn't one coming?

The reason is clear enough. I believe that our failure to eradicate cancer is due largely to another myth. This myth has been the point of origin for virtually all cancer research. In other words, the belief that has driven doctors for decades in research labs around the world is a myth.

The myth is that there is a cure for cancer. The myth is the belief in a "silver bullet" that will single handedly rid the world of this unbearable disease. The mainstream medical community's failure to conquer cancer is directly connected with its reluctance to abandon belief in this myth.

I don't believe that we will ever find "a cure." Cancer presents us with a dizzying array of variations. Couple that with the unique physiology of each and every patient and it doesn't take a genius to recognize that there will never be a "magic pill" that can cover all of those variables.

If we ever hope to become cancer free, we must embrace reality over mythology. We must remove our heads from the sand and seek a viewpoint that provides a clear vision of the situation. The right vantage is vital, because it will help us avoid unnecessary setback and heartbreak.

As I set out to write this book, my goal is to provide you with information that will demystify cancer. I want to empower you to make choices that will help you overcome the cancer challenge. Though I know of no magical cure to cancer, I can assure you of one thing. There is hope.

My father and I have treated over 100,000 patients for over 60 years combined. Our work has not been in vain. We have identified therapies that promise a benefit but don't work at all. We have also identified many effective therapies and a treatment approach that can position people for full recovery.

The thrust of this book is twofold. First, it should serve to debunk the two primary myths surrounding cancer. Cancer is a very real disease and it is important that we approach it with a hopeful and realistic perspective. We will examine why the mainstream approach to cancer treatment has become what it is today. More importantly, we will take an honest look at the successes and shortcomings of the three mainstream treatment methods: chemotherapy, radiation, and surgery.

Second, the book should serve to explain the "total care" approach and the spectrum of choice that lies within it. We need to develop a proper understanding of immunotherapy and the self-healing concept. We need to understand how important the body, mind, and spirit are in the recovery process. We will examine the highlights from the body of research on natural anticancer agents compiled at the Oasis of Hope Hospital.

Make no mistake, I'm not claiming that my father and I are the discoverers of these effective cancer therapies. I'm not going to pretend that we invented the body, mind, and spirit approach. What we have done differently for the last 40 years is implement new therapies quickly. The wheels of change turn painfully slow in the mainstream medical community, principally because there is so much money tied up in conventional treatment methods. Many doctors find it difficult to apply new therapies that medical journals have indicated are beneficial and equally difficult to steer away from therapies that studies demonstrate are not effective. So much beneficial research lays dormant on the shelves of medical libraries.

At the Oasis of Hope, we are decades ahead of the mainstream community because of our willingness to embrace change. It is the insights from almost half a century of experience that I wish to share with you. My desire is that this book fills you with tremendous hope and helps you to make some informed decisions.

# CHAPTER TWO

## A Need For Change

Have you ever noticed the reluctance of the male species to stop an automobile and ask for directions? My wife has. There must be a genetic switch somewhere that predisposes men to stubbornness in this area. I would rather endure an hour of unanesthetized kneecap surgery than admit I don't know where I'm going. Even when I'm forced to acknowledge that I'm lost I won't stop and ask for help. I will put my ear to the ground, or examine the lichen on a nearby tree to determine which direction I should go. Then I will clamber back into the car and grunt like a caveman, "Water that way. We go north." Sadly, my unwillingness to admit defeat always yields the same result. We arrive late.

The medical community has behaved in much the same way when it comes to the treatment of cancer. The lack of significant reduction in the incidence of cancer and the mortality rate of cancer are clear indicators that doctors are lost and moving in the wrong direction.

The 20th century will go down in history as the era of scientific breakthrough and technological advance. It is hard to believe that we started out the 1900s without electricity, telephones, automobiles, and computers. The medical field was profoundly impacted by the scientific and technological revolutions. Scientists developed an arsenal of pharmaceuticals designed to address just about every pathogen. Meanwhile, new technology like lasers, 3-D imaging devices, and fiber optic cameras assisted physicians in the field. The results of these advances have been impressive.

Acute medicine is at the top of its game, for one. Doctors are able to save life and limb in ways never before thought possible. If Humpty Dumpty had been brought to a modern day trauma center, he would have been put back together in no time at all.

In addition, once complex medical procedures like angioplasty and open-heart surgery have become routine. People don't fret as much as they used to when they go under the knife. Technology has made the operating room a much more controlled environment than before.

Finally, diseases like polio, smallpox, and tuberculosis have nearly been eliminated in developed countries. Yet, there is a danger in all of this good news. The advances of medicine in the 20th century have led many people into a false sense of security.

Society's overconfidence in doctors has caused many to adopt a cavalier attitude toward personal health. Many people live however they want, eat whatever they want, and disregard any responsibility for their own health. These people hold the erroneous belief that the doctor can fix every problem.

*Then, there is cancer...*

I'm sure that when the incidence of cancer began to rise in the first half of the 20th century, doctors were confident that this was just another epidemic that would meet its demise at the hands of modern medicine. As the century progressed, I can imagine the horror with which they realized the truth. I believe that many doctors recognized by the 1950s that they were dealing with an enemy of gargantuan proportions. After all, one out of every four deaths in the United States is attributed to cancer. These doctors did what anyone would do when threatened with such terrifying opposition: they went in search of a weapon to kill it.

Scientists were so sure that they could find the cure if they had proper funding. They made such a convincing case that they were able to gain federal support. In 1971, President Richard Nixon signed the National Cancer Act[1] to dedicate part of the national budget to cancer research through the National Cancer Institute.

Unfortunately, the incidence and mortality rates of cancer have increased every year since. So, what has been the benefit of all that research funding? I'll tell you. It has taught us two important lessons. First, it has taught us that we cannot buy the cure to cancer. Second, it has taught us that we need to search for the cause instead of the cure.

Yet, mainstream medicine continues to ignore these lessons. Scientists continue to spend obscene amounts of money every year searching for the "silver bullet," and doctors continue to rely on the orthodox treatments of surgery, radiation, and chemotherapy. Let's take a look at how those treatments became the industry standards and why the medical community is so reluctant to abandon them.

Most medical historians will agree that the surgical treatment of cancer began around the turn of the century. A key historical figure of the time was William Halsted, considered the father of surgery in the United States. In Halsted's day, the treatment of breast cancer was extreme, often involving the removal of the entire breast.[2]  In part this was because Halsted hypothesized that cancer grew by spreading "tentacles" out from a centralized area into the rest of the body. Nobody imagined that carcinogenic cells traveled via the blood stream.[3]  When a cancer spread to surrounding organs, it was believed that the "tentacles" had grown in those directions.

This theory became the foundation of oncological surgery. Therefore, the best course of action seemed obvious. Doctors felt that removing any tissue that could contain the cancer's "tentacles" would give a patient the best chances for survival. The most common of these surgeries was the radical mastectomy. These procedures were disturbing and often seriously compromised the patient's quality of life. Yet, the philosophy of radical surgery for breast cancer was soon applied to other cancers. Many of the surgeries performed during that era were absolutely nightmarish.

Relief appeared to come in 1910, when evidence came to light that cancerous cells travel via the blood stream. The process was referred to as metastasis. Though metastasis made the disease even more elusive, many hoped that the gruesome practice of radical surgery would fall by the wayside, as Halsted's foundational hypothesis crumbled. Yet, it continued.

In 1964, the first comparitive study between radical surgery and conservative surgery of breast cancer was conducted. The study clearly demonstrated that the patients treated with conservative surgery had a life expectancy equal to or greater than those treated with radical surgery. Yet, many doctors continue to perform these drastic surgeries today without any "scientific" foundation to support the decision to do so.

How is it possible that almost a century after the discovery of metastasis, the medical community has failed to abandon a surgical practice that is grounded on a blatantly false hypothesis? What justification is there to continue this practice when clinical studies prove that such a course of action is absolutely unnecessary?[4] These are good questions, but radical surgery is not the only cancer treatment we should examine carefully.

Almost half a century has passed since radiation therapy was fully embraced as an orthodox treatment method by the mainstream medical community. In the early years, there was hope that radiation would prove to be highly effective. Yet, in that time it has proved to be of little use. As physicians met with failure they chose to apply increasingly aggressive doses, rather than abandon the practice. The results of this decision were frightening. Patients were literally "burned" in the treatment process, often sustaining irreversible damage that left them disabled. To make matters worse, the intense side-effects of severe nausea and general malaise seriously reduced the patient's quality of life.

The aggressive application of chemotherapy did not improve matters for cancer patients either. A major study into the effectiveness of chemotherapy by Dr. Ulrich Abel revealed the ineffectiveness of the treatment. In the study, Dr. Abel affirms that there is no evidence that the vast majority of cancer treatments with cytotoxic drugs (chemotherapy) exert any kind of positive influence as far as life expectancy or quality of life are concerned.[5]

Again, failure has driven chemotherapists to administer increasingly aggressive dosages and to use considerably more intense cytotoxic substances. Of the three orthodox treatment methods, chemotherapy may be the most destructive. In most cases, patients feel like they are dying. The nausea and vomiting are often severe enough to require hospitalization. Chemotherapy patients suffer the loss of hair, appetite, and the energy needed to battle disease. I cannot tell you how many patients I have spoken with who would rather die than continue with the therapy. It disturbs me that people would actually prefer to live with cancer and a prognosis of certain death, than to suffer the experience of chemotherapy. It is clear that many view the therapy as a fate worse than death.

My brother, Dr. José Ernesto Contreras. is a clinical oncologist. He shared my disappointment stating, "It is really frustrating to see how little we have been able to advance ... against cancer. I have treated more than 40,000 patients, most of them in the late stages of cancer, and I can't say that more than 15 percent of them responded positively to an orthodox therapy. Only about 40 percent received the benefit of temporary remission, or the alleviation of suffering. The remaining 60 percent felt little or no reduction in their suffering. I can only remember a few patients whose lives were significantly prolonged by the aggressive treatments now available. In most cases studied, we had to conclude that the remedy was worse than the disease."

My brother and I are not alone. In 1969, Dr. Hardin James of the University of California at Berkeley reported, at an American Cancer Society conference, that patients not subjected to aggressive therapies had a longer life expectancy, than those who underwent aggressive treatment. In 1986, Dr. Bailar III and Elaine Smith reported that patients with lung cancer who refused treatment experienced a longer life expectancy and a better quality of life than those who received treatment.[6] In 1988, Dr. Abel reported that patients suffering from pancreatic cancer who received a placebo treatment lived longer and better. Dr. Bailar III, upon evaluating the results of cancer therapies between 1950 and 1980, rated them to be a "qualified failure." These men and women are not joking when they assert that both the treatment methods and the direction of research must change.

If surgery, radiation, and chemotherapy have been so unsuccessful, why is it that mainstream medicine has not rejected them? In other branches of science and industry, worthless things are rejected and then substituted by things that have value. Nevertheless, in the struggle against cancer this has not been the case. The governmental authorities, scientific community, and pharmaceutical monopolies have placed serious obstacles in the path of new ideas. Alternative therapies, many of which have been proven effective, have been ridiculed, pushed aside, and prohibited. These therapies do not deteriorate the patient's quality of life. It is well known that patients suffering from many malignancies live longer and better if the orthodox treatments (surgery, radiation, and chemotherapy) are not applied.

Just a couple of years ago, a renowned oncologist came to visit my father. He explained that he had cancer and was looking for someone to treat him. My father asked him, "Why not take the chemotherapy that you have prescribed to your patients over the past 30 years?" The doctor responded, "But this is me we are talking about Ernesto!" This cancer specialist's experience treating thousands of cancer patients had taught him that chemotherapy alone was not going to cure him. He came to my father looking for an integrative approach.

I am convinced that the real and practical value of the aggressive use of surgery, radiation, and chemotherapy is very limited. Therefore, it should be the obligation of leading oncologists and physicians to investigate new and alternative treatments. Only then can we hope to find more effective, less aggressive, and less toxic treatments. Only then can we hope to prolong the lives of cancer patients and maintain the quality of their lives as well.

I can assure you there are no silver bullets. Conventional therapies such as surgery, radiation, and chemotherapy can succeed in the destruction of malignant cells, but they still fail to address the root cause of the cancer. That is why doctors see so many patients whose initial response to conventional treatment was positive, back in the hospital months or years later with stage IV cancer. Doctors need to abandon the silver bullet methodology and use a multi-disciplinary approach that meets the physical, emotional, and spiritual needs of the patient.

The Oasis of Hope is perceived, by doctors and patients, here and abroad, as an alternative hospital. The truth is that it is more, much more than that. In the summer of 2002, at a health convention in New York, I was invited to participate in a debate about cancer therapies. As you can imagine, the bulk of the public was biased against anything that even smelled orthodox. In fact, some local oncologists had voiced their opposition to the convention so the organizers invited them for this discussion to avoid frictions that could cancel the event. I applauded their effort and was gladly surprised that these guys even showed up.

The panel consisted of physicians and practitioners of orthodox and alternative therapies. In the heat of the battle, I confronted the orthodox oncologists with the facts stated in this chapter, cheers! To the surprise of many, I also criticized the alternative practitioners who believe that even the most complicated of cases could be resolved with green juices, a couple of enemas, and a load of vitamins, jeers! Here we were discussing the fate of cancer patients and not one practitioner on the alternative side was a cancer specialist, except me. My candid comments got the attention of the crowd, which came to life with a barrage of comments and questions.

A frustrated member of the organizing committee, by now sorry he had invited me to be a member of the panel, stood up and asked me, Dr. Contreras, "Which is it, do you practice alternative medicine or orthodox medicine?" A hush fell over the audience. They were sitting on the edges of their seats. I was sure that more than one was aiming tomatoes (organic, I hoped) at my head. "I do not want to practice orthodox or alternative medicine," I said. "I only want to practice good medicine. I use any and all means to help my patients so that, God willing, they may enjoy life for a long time." The tension eased and people relaxed back in their chairs. One in the back started clapping, then another one, then a few more. I didn't deserve the standing ovation; patients deserve it for being so courageous. I am very selective about what treatment I will offer my patients but it is not the type of therapy that matters to me. Even the most non-toxic approach can be used wrongly to the detriment of a patient. It is how and why a therapy is used that really matters. Will it improve my patient's chances of survival without jeopardizing quality of life? Would I use the same approach, chemotherapy or laetrile, if I or any of my children was the patient?

My father and I have championed the multi-disciplinary approach for decades. When it comes to cancer, doctors must consider every option. There is a host of treatments that achieve tumor destruction without compromising the patient's quality of life. Yet, I have found that our beliefs have placed us between a rock and a hard place. On the one hand, orthodox doctors have spoken out against us because of our use of natural therapies. At the same time, alternative doctors have lashed out at us for our non-aggressive use of surgery, radiation, and chemotherapy.

Our motive to branch away from the mainstream has not been to gain popularity. I, like my father before me, am driven by my concern for the well being of my patients. Thus, I refuse to rule out any therapy option. If it will improve the patient's quality of life and his prognosis, I will use it. Aside from our choice of therapies, the emotional and spiritual support we integrate into our treatment program is the differentiating aspect of our hospital.

Doctors need to get back to the art of medicine, which begins with building a relationship with the patient. Science must come second as a tool to guide physicians. Technology is a plus but human touch is vital. Knowing and listening to patients will often uncover what blood tests and x-rays can't find. Doctors need to treat the whole person. That means finding the physical imbalances that cause breakdowns in the immune system. It also means addressing the emotional and spiritual issues that depress the immune system. These things open the door to cancer.

Remember, that part of the problem has been our search for the cure instead of the cause. We have wasted precious time treating the disease instead of the patient. So, what does it look like when doctors treat the patient instead of the disease? Let's take a look.

# Chapter Three

## *The Road Less Traveled*

There are some words a person never forgets. I'll never forget the first time my wife said, "I love you." I'll never forget where I was when my first child said, "papa." I'll never forget the last words my father said to me. These and many more are etched into the tablets of my mind forever.

"A doctor should never tell a patient, 'there is nothing more I can do for you.' A doctor can always serve a patient, even if it is just holding his hand through a tough night." I can still picture my father's face as he spoke these words. His eyes burned with a passionate focus. My father never lost sight of the human side of his patients. His love for people grew into a vision of a hospital that would provide care for the whole patient; body, mind, and spirit.

In the early years, he and his contemporaries were fascinated by the wave of technological advancement in the medical field. Yet, for many of his colleagues, the fascination became unhealthy. As they grew more dependent upon new technology, they cultivated an increasingly objective distance from their patients. Many of these physicians began to believe that the wisest decisions were those that were unclouded by emotional attachment.

So, while the rest of the pack worked hard to establish a healthy professional distance from their patients, my dad began to spend more time with his. He wanted to know his patients on a personal level. He needed to find out if any emotional or spiritual stress were contributing to his patients' illnesses.

In the mornings, he behaved like a conventional doctor. He prescribed lab work, x-rays, and medication. In the afternoons, he behaved quite unconventionally. He gathered his patients together to talk, sing, laugh, and pray. He offered words of encouragement and the warm hug of a man who cared. He began to combine sound medicine supported with intentional emotional and spiritual support. It was this that first caused patients to begin to refer to the Contreras Hospital as an "oasis of hope."

Today, the Oasis of Hope Hospital is a high-tech medical/surgical facility. The hospital employs cutting-edge technology like digital CT scanners and state-of-the-art touch screen ventilators. Doctors have access to electronic medical files through a wireless local area network, which allows them to access patient records on palmtops or tablet PCs. Patients surf the web on broadband workstations and keep in touch with loved ones via digital telephone lines. However, the hospital had very humble beginnings. This was due, in part, to my father's struggle to break free from the confines of the mainstream medical community that was rapidly driving a wedge between physician and patient.

In 1939, my father began his career in medicine. As a recent graduate of the army medical school in Mexico City, he expressed his desire to specialize in a new field of medicine, pathology. Encouraged by his professors, he applied for an internship at Boston's Children Hospital, an extension of Harvard University. He was accepted. The challenges there were memorable, but they were nothing like the ones to come.

When he returned to Mexico, more intense challenges were waiting. The army sent him to the city of Tijuana, located at the northernmost point along the coastline of the Baja peninsula. What made the assignment so overwhelming was the scarcity of pathologists in those days. My father was the first in that region of the world.

Hospitals across the border in San Diego were desperate for the services of a qualified pathologist and were quick to contact my father. For the first few years of his practice, he would work in San

Diego in the mornings and in Tijuana in the afternoons. He was working harder than he ever had.

What exactly is a pathologist, you ask? A pathologist is the specialist that analyzes blood and tissue samples to determine what type of pathology (illness) is present. For example, it is the pathologist who determines whether a tumor biopsy is benign (non-cancerous) or malignant (cancerous). During those early years, my father spent hours at his microscope each day examining tissue given to him for analysis from doctors. He began to notice that many of the organs that doctors were removing were healthy and that there were far too many unnecessary surgeries being performed. He knew these doctors well and he knew that they had the best of intentions, yet he felt there must be a way to improve the diagnostic process and thereby reduce the number of unnecessary surgeries being performed.

People were excited about his ideas and he was offered a full-time position at Mercy Hospital in San Diego, California. The job came complete with immigration documents and a probability of U.S. citizenship. It was a tempting offer, to say the least, but my father declined it. In his heart he felt called to make a contribution to his home country. So, he decided to get out from behind the microscope and start treating patients with the goal of improving the diagnostic process.

There are moments in life that change you as a person, that alter the direction you choose to travel forever. For my father, that moment occurred in 1963 when Cecile Hoffman came to see him. Cecile was a cancer patient. She had suffered several grueling rounds of chemotherapy and had been told there was no hope. Determined not to give up, she looked into alternative therapies. She found one.

Cecile had traveled to Canada to acquire the substance laetrile but she wanted to find a doctor close to home to treat her. It was this desire that brought her to my father. She asked him if he would be willing to oversee her laetrile treatments. In the blink of an eye, my father's experience with alternative therapies began. He never looked back.

My father admitted that his hopes for Cecile were not high, given the prognosis offered by the doctors she had seen. However, the treatments gave her hope and she appeared to be getting stronger. As the laetrile treatment progressed, my father became absolutely astonished. Here was a woman, who had undergone conventional therapies to no avail, who was given a death sentence, who was getting better. In the end, my father had no choice but to acknowledge that Cecile Hoffman had completely overcome cancer.

Cecile went on to start an organization called "Cancer Victims and Friends," which birthed the "Cancer Control Society." The organization held its first seminar in the backyard of her home featuring Dr. Ernesto Contreras, Sr., as the keynote speaker. As a result, my father began to receive floods of patients who, like Cecile, had been given no hope after chemotherapy failed to help them. Word of mouth spread and my mother and father were faced with a dilemma. The consultation office was too small and what would they do with the patients who needed to be hospitalized?

The Oasis of Hope Hospital actually started in our house. My mother always had a way of finding solutions to every challenge. When it became apparent that a patient my father was seeing needed hospital care, she would send us children across the street to stay with neighbors. Presto! Our rooms became patient rooms. She was the first Oasis nurse and administrator.

In 1966, my parents went on a trip that followed the route taken by the Apostle Paul on his missionary travels. When the tour guide discovered that my father was a physician, he took him to see an ancient healing center in Pergamum. Ernesto's eyes were opened as he learned that the healing process in those days always involved the combination of physical, emotional, and spiritual therapies. At that moment, he realized that the problem with modern medicine was that doctors had forgotten that a person has a body, mind, and spirit. The focus had become the illness in the body.

Embracing the vision of treating the whole person, my father began his mission to improve the quality of the physical, emotional, and spiritual care of his patients. He envisioned a facility that could provide quality medical services coupled with emotional and spiritual support services. That vision is the Oasis of Hope Hospital.

To this day, the hospital is guided by his vision. We continue to blend science, compassion, and faith in all that we do. We believe that the needs of the patient should determine what therapies should be offered. We continue to incorporate a wide variety of treatment modalities, from the manufactured to the natural, from the conventional to the holistic. Yet, for all the bells and whistles that change has brought about in our facilities, the guiding principles have remained constant.

After all, everything starts and finishes with philosophy. Think about it. It doesn't matter what field a person is in, the highest degree is a Doctor of Philosophy. There are Ph.D.'s in immunology, anthropology, mathematics, and literature. That is because philosophy shapes everything you do.

The philosophy my father established at Oasis can be defined by two guiding principles he gave to his medical staff:

1. Do no harm. Never compromise your patient's quality of life.
2. Love your patient as yourself.

So simple yet profound. If a physician contemplates these principles each and every day, it will challenge him to find the most effective treatment with the least amount of negative side effects.

Unfortunately, oncologists often lose sight of the general condition and well-being of the patient, because so much of their attention is focused and directed toward the destruction of the tumor. Modern doctors can, and often do, unintentionally compromise the quality of a person's life in their blind determination to eliminate disease.

The doctors at the Oasis of Hope Hospital embrace a different focus. Bound by oath to do no harm and to love our patients, we only offer therapies that have the potential to improve the patient's health without compromising quality of life. If we determine that juice

therapy will benefit a patient, we offer it. If we believe that chemotherapy will benefit a patient, we offer it. However, we will always
apply a therapy in a form that will avoid the negative side effects that
deteriorate quality of life.

Has the Oasis philosophy and total care approach really helped
people? Read the patient testimonials on our Internet site
(*www.oasisofhope.com*) if you are curious. Our patients share their
cancer experience and explain how Oasis helped them overcome
cancer. Want hard data? All right, let's take a look at the numbers.

In 1981, my father conducted a retrospective study to document the five-year survival rates of our cancer patients. It is important to note that 95 percent of these patients came to us with stage IV
cancers after conventional therapy had failed to help them. Stage IV
is the most advanced stage of cancer. The disease reaches stage IV
when the cancer has spread to other parts of the body from the primary site. Once patients reach stage IV, conventional doctors gen-
erally tell them that there is no chance for survival. This is why they
come to Oasis. They are desperate for hope.

These patients were treated by our total care approach and the
Oasis overall five-year survival rate for all types of cancer was 30
percent. We also noted that 86 percent of our patients outlived their
prognosis and reported an improvement in their quality of life.

Lung, breast, colon, and prostate cancers are some of the most
common in our world today. For this reason, we choose to study the
effectiveness of our treatment program with stage IV cancers of these
four types. In Table 1 (see page 33), we compared our results against
those from clinical trials with conventional therapies.

Compared to conventional therapies, the treatment program at
the Oasis of Hope Hospital yielded dramatically better results. What
makes these numbers even more astounding to me is the difference
between the two patient groups. The patients in the conventional
group who survived had not been through previous treatments that
would have deteriorated their natural defenses and robbed them of
vital energy. They had a fresh start. However, the patients in the

Oasis group were those who had suffered the ravages of surgery, radiation, or chemotherapy. Yet, we were still able to help them.

**TABLE 1. SURVIVAL RATES FOR STAGE IV CANCERS**

| Type of cancer Distant[1] | Number of patients | 5 yr. survival rate (%) Oasis | Conventional[2] |
|---|---|---|---|
| Lung Cancer | 200 | 30% | 3% |
| Breast Cancer | 130 | 39% | 23% |
| Colon Cancer | 150 | 30% | 9% |
| Prostate Cancer | 600 | 86% | 34% |

1. Distant: A malignant cancer that has spread to parts of the body remote from the primary tumor either by direct extension or by discontinuous metastasis to distant organs, tissues, or via the lymphatic system to distant lymph nodes.
2. Source: American Cancer Society. Cancer Facts & Figures 2003.

Cancer is a challenge like no other because this killer has an uncanny ability to mutate and resist adversity, like pests to pesticides, or bacteria to antibiotics. Thus, the malignancies of the 70s are not the malignancies of today. Cervical cancer used to be a "regional" tumor that invaded the pelvis but "never" spread beyond it. Now, it is not infrequent to find liver or even lung metastasis from it. The aggressiveness of almost all malignancies has increased. Where almost all prostate cancers used to be "low grade," very often we admit patients with extremely aggressive prostate tumors that are refractive to any kind of treatment. The age at diagnosis has dramatically diminished. While in the 70s most of our patients were in their 70s, in the new millennium most patients are in their 40s.

At the Oasis of Hope, we have made pertinent adjustment to keep the "playing field" leveled. I would love to tell you that we are getting much better results that we did twenty years ago. I can't.

While it continues to be true that malignant cells cannot become resistant to cyanide, the active ingredient of amygdalin, tumors have become more aggressive. I will tell you that in my opinion, to be able to get results today, with how much more difficult cancer is than it was thirty years ago, I am very happy.

Taking all of this into account, we have been very proactive in research and development, not only in the therapeutical realm but also in the data-managing arena. A new and comprehensive software was developed specifically for Oasis to assist the research team to evaluate results.

We are proud of the results we have presented here from prospective clinical trials done in the 70s. I wish that obstacles would not have been put in the way for publication in medical journals, but I am confident in the future that we will be able to share our results with the medical community. Our administrative and medical teams have worked hard to obtain fresh data that represents results of the new cancer era.

We began accumulating data with our new research software in 2001 and now have results, supported with hard data of three-year survival rates for patients with the most common cancers.

In spite of the fact that the average age of our patients is much lower now (50s vs. 70s) and that these tumors are much more aggressive, our preliminary results are quite encouraging. These numbers are pretty much what they will be at the five-year point. All the patients included in the study were diagnosed with stage IV malignancies and conventional therapies failed them. These are patients that literally were expected to live between weeks and a few months.

Of the patients that came with breast cancer, 59 percent are alive after three years of Oasis therapy; 31 percent of patients suffering from colon cancer with liver metastasis are alive when life expectancy is really only four months; 33 percent of our patients with inoperable lung cancer are still alive after three years of Oasis therapy. Do not forget that 98 percent of patients diagnosed with stage IV lung cancer die within twelve months regardless of the treatment; 67

percent of our patients with prostatic cancer in stage IV are alive while, according to the ACS, only 8 percent are alive after five years.

These are very encouraging results, but we are not resting in our laurels; we are committed to stay the course and give cancer a black eye.

I have come to the conclusion that my father knew what he was doing when he chose the road less traveled many years ago. His choice has made a world of difference to many people in the last forty years. So, what exactly does the treatment program at the Oasis of Hope Hospital look like? Are you curious? Keep reading.

# CHAPTER FOUR

## Good Medicine

In 2003, when the space shuttle Columbia disintegrated in the atmosphere upon re-entry, I watched news footage of its brightly-lit pieces hurtling across the sky in absolute horror. Yet what struck me most about the incident was the search for a cause. In the days that followed the tragedy, various NASA experts formed a host of hypotheses. Many of the things that could have caused the disaster were small intricate pieces of the shuttle. The importance of the smallest part became abundantly clear to all those who followed the story.

I wonder if we can even imagine the intensity of the safety precautions NASA engineers and mechanics follow. It takes millions of parts to build a space shuttle and every one is of critical importance. I'm sure that each and every part is checked and tested thoroughly, from the biggest piece of framework to the smallest rivet. If everything is to work properly, nothing can be overlooked.

And so it is with the dismantling of cancer. If the healing process is to work properly, nothing can be overlooked: not the body, not the mind, and not the spirit. That has been one of my two main points thus far. We must see the body, mind, and spirit as three critical components in the healing process. To ignore any of those components can spell disaster.

Doctors must also be open to alternatives when conventional medicine alone offers no benefit. That is my second main point. What do those individual components look like at the Oasis of Hope? Let's take a look.

When people seeking medical help hear the word "alternative" they immediately conjure up visions of some shady looking character selling miracle-grow hair tonic from the back of some horse-drawn cart. It is true that there are some "physicians" of questionable authenticity in the world today, as well as some "alternative" medical practices of dubious quality. In sharp contrast to "fly by night" operations, the Oasis of Hope medical staff carry truly impressive credentials, from some of the finest medical institutions around the world. Every aspect of our medical treatment program is methodic, precise, scientifically sound and comprehensive in nature. Oasis of Hope is a proud member of the American Hospital Association and enjoys the reputation as being the finest treatment center in the northwest of Mexico.

Though our focus is on the total care of the patient and not merely the illness, we have not lessened the intensity of our medical practice. We use all that modern technology has to offer to help us determine the true physical needs of the patient and we firmly believe in employing only those practices that adhere to strict international standards. The medical component of the Oasis of Hope program divides easily into the following five segments: examination and diagnostic tests, detoxification of the body, stimulation of the immune system, application of antitumor agents, and alteration of lifestyle.

## Examination and Diagnostic Tests

I have always loved tennis. Ever since the days of the Borg-McEnroe rivalry I have loved the game. When I first began to play, I was like most people. I hit the ball hard and it seldom went where I wanted it to go. The competitor in me wanted to improve, so I worked at it. I did improve to a point but there were areas of my game that never seemed to go beyond a certain plateau. Then I went to a tennis coach.

I remember stepping onto the court ready to rally back and forth and have him explain the finer points of the game. Instead, he set up the camcorder and we spent the next hour filming me hitting every imaginable stroke from every imaginable angle. When the hour was up, he packed up the camera, shook my hand, and dropped off the face of the planet for a week.

When he set up the next appointment at my home, I ran out with a tape measure and determined that there was no way we could play tennis in the driveway. He sat in my living room, popped the tape he had filmed in the VCR, and deconstructed every aspect of my tennis stroke, from the grip to the turn of my hips. I realized that he was going to tailor-make his instruction to fit my specific issues as a tennis player. I have never been happier to write a check in my entire life.

When doctors at Oasis first meet a patient, they try to find out everything they can in an effort to tailor-make an appropriate treatment course. Patients are asked to bring all medical records from previous treatments. They must provide all medication prescriptions, laboratory reports, x-rays, CT scans, MRI reports, and radiological reports that have been generated since the original diagnosis. The medical team then conducts a comprehensive study to verify the patient's condition and confirm if the previous diagnosis is correct. This study is comprised of four parts: a clinical history, an oncological examination, a series of blood tests and urinalyses, and a radiological examination.

The formation of an accurate clinical history involves more than the simple collection of medical records. Oasis physicians always sit down with a patient and conduct a thorough interview in order to construct a far more accurate picture than the pile of medical documentation alone can generate. There is an old saying among doctors that if you "listen to a patient long enough, he will tell you exactly what is causing his illness." Old sayings become old sayings because there is a good measure of truth in them.

In this interview, the doctors ask about the patient's family history of illness, allergies to medications, general physical state, and general emotional state. In addition, the doctors will try to determine if there are any aspects of the patient's lifestyle that may be affecting the patient's health. Every doctor at Oasis understands that it is here that the vital bond between doctor and patient begins to form. When people are sick they want to know that they are being listened to and that their thoughts and feelings matter.

The oncological examination is a lot like a physical exam but the intent is completely different. Oasis doctors have been trained to look for specific conditions related to cancer. The doctors take note of these conditions and search for anything else that previous doctors may have overlooked.

Complete blood panels and urinalysis are performed throughout the treatment process. Initially, Oasis doctors use these tests to determine how well the patient's immune system is functioning, and how well critical organs are functioning prior to receiving treatment. However, as treatment progresses, tumor markers are taken periodically to measure the patient's response to the program.

The radiological examination involves a number of x-rays, CT scans, and ultrasounds. Our doctors use these tests to determine the extent to which the cancer has progressed. However, these tests are also performed periodically during a patient's stay. This helps the team of doctors gauge whether the cancer is progressing or digressing. The continuing tests also help doctors identify sites of possible metastasis.

Once all of this diagnostic information has been collected, it is integrated into an electronic patient file. A team of specialists discusses the patient's case at a biweekly medical board meeting. In this way, each patient benefits from the expertise of a diverse group of physicians, who bring their own unique training and varied experience to the table. It is in these board meetings that a patient's treatment program is customized to address the specific needs of the patient. At each subsequent meeting the team of doctors looks at new diagnostic information, re-evaluates the patient's case, and makes adjustments as necessary.

## Detoxification of the Body

I remember an art exhibit I visited once at a museum in San Diego, California. I have always been a fan of the impressionists and there were quite a few of Monet's paintings at this particular show. The pieces were breathtaking, from beautiful garden scenes to explosions of color along the French countryside. Then, I stepped into the next room. There, in a corner, was a painting of his I was not familiar with at all.

It was a small painting, a view of the river Seine and Paris in the distance. From the left of the painting a thin stretch of riverbank crept into the foreground, with a little ramshackle shed sagging low to the earth. What struck me about the painting was the color. Unlike the majority of Monet's work, which is a celebration of the love affair between color and light, this painting was a mass of grays, browns, and black. Factories belched smoke into the air along the Parisian horizon and the river seemed to be a slog of dirt and waste.

The painting, I found out, was Monet's reaction to the industrial revolution in France. As I drew nearer I could see that the paint was smeared thick and violent. The painter's disgust was evident in the work. It is no secret that our drive to produce has dirtied the planet to a horrifying extent.

Everyone comes in contact with toxic agents on a daily basis. Toxins are present in the food we eat, the water we drink, and the air we breathe. Many of these toxins are carcinogens, meaning they poison the body in such a way as to make it very susceptible to cancer. These carcinogens are present in carpet, paint, plastics, and just about every man-made material ever manufactured.

So, our bodies constantly endure the stress of battling and eliminating these substances. Yet, cancer patients have it even worse. Not only are their bodies taxed with the task of combating these carcinogens, but many of the conventional medications they are subjected to flood the body with even more toxic agents. This is why the second segment of the Oasis of Hope's medical treatment program is so vital.

After the diagnostic examination, each Oasis patient begins a mild detoxification program, designed to rid the body of many of the harmful substances stored within it. This serves two purposes. First, it helps the body to receive optimal benefit from the therapies we offer. Second, it helps to restore proper function to the immune system.

The detoxification process involves the use of intravenous solutions of vitamin C, potassium, immuno-modulators, polarizing agents, and chelating agents. The combined effect of these substances is to gently pull stored toxins out of the tissue they are stored in and introduce them back into the blood stream where the body can effectively eliminate them. The process also involves coffee or tea enemas to stimulate liver function, and high colonics to alleviate intestinal blockages and promote proper bowel function. All of these things are fundamental to effective toxin elimination. The results are amazing.

When the detoxification process is finished, patients often comment that they feel better and stronger than they have felt in months. The Oasis doctors know that the healthier the body is, the better equipped it is to combat cancer.

## Stimulation of the Immune System

I watched a television documentary series recently on the Navy Seals. The series followed a group of candidates through the grueling training and testing process one must endure to become a member of the Navy Seals. I have never seen human beings willingly subject themselves to the kind of physical punishment these men did. They ran until they were sick... but they had to run more to pass. They swam until water rushed into their lungs... but they had to force the water out and finish unassisted to pass. They swam in extreme cold and then stood on the deck of a submarine in their trunks, shivering until their teeth chattered... but they had to get back in the water over and over again to pass. The men who failed the program were athletic, driven, and courageous. The men who passed the program defy description. They are the toughest fighting machines on the face of the earth and the best the Navy has to offer, no question. If I were going to war, I'd want men like that on my side. Wouldn't you?

The reality is that dismantling cancer *is* a war. The battlefield is inside of us, which is why the third segment of the Oasis medical treatment program is critical. If the body is engaging in an act of war, it needs to be as ready as a Navy Seal. The Oasis immunotherapy program prepares a body for internal combat. It provides the body with all the vital resources needed to bolster the immune system. The immunotherapy program is comprised of the following three components: juice therapy, nutrition therapy, and Vitamin/Mineral/Enzyme (VME) therapy.

Juice therapy is simply the daily intake of organic juices, mostly carrot and green juices. Oasis doctors prescribe a juice regimen initially to detoxify the body and then modify the regimen to boost the immune system. The hospital uses certified organically grown vegetables that are toxin free and loaded with all of the vitamins, minerals, and phytochemicals the body needs to repair itself.

One of the best ways to provide healing resources to the body is through foods. Unfortunately, the typical patient adheres to the Standard American Diet (SAD). It should not come as a shock to anyone to learn that this diet is low in fiber and high in fat, white flour, sugar, preservatives, cholesterol, pesticides, antibiotics, and hormones. All of these things are known to inhibit proper function of the immune system.

At the Oasis of Hope, patients enjoy lots of nutrient-dense fruits and vegetables that strengthen the immune system. These foods are organically grown and free of the preservatives, pesticides, and antibiotics that can depress the immune system. In addition, the Oasis of Hope diet is high in fiber, promoting proper bowel function and waste elimination. Finally, the food is delicious!

Tasty and nutritious foods are not an extra part of the Oasis program. These foods are fundamental. The reason why we use food as medicine is because the nutrients in food are more bioavailable than the nutrients packaged in drugs and nutraceuticals. This means that the body can process the nutrients more efficiently and put them to work quickly. This is not true of many vitamin products on the market today.

While it is true organic juices and foods are the best source of the essential nutrients the immune system needs to function at optimal levels, I strongly believe in supplementing these therapies with vitamins, minerals, and enzymes. Organic juices and foods can provide adequate nutrition for a healthy person, but the person whose immune system has been compromised needs more resources than diet alone can provide. This is why the Oasis VME therapy is the last piece of the immunotherapy program.

The vitamin and mineral solutions used at Oasis provide powerful antioxidants that are instrumental in the detoxification process. Oasis patients also take oral supplements that provide many of the antioxidants and phytochemicals the immune system needs to battle disease effectively. The combination of these three therapies can transform the body's immune system into an incredible fighting machine. Chapter six will explain immunotherapy in more depth.

*Application of Antitumor Agents*

If you follow the sport of hockey at all you will know that the NHL has changed considerably in the last twenty years. A steady influx of players from overseas has increased the speed and finesse with which the game is played. Players like Sergei Fedorov, Peter Forsberg, and Teemu Selanne have helped to take goal scoring to new heights. Yet, there is a player on every team whose job is as old as the league: the enforcer.

Every team has to have a player whose job it is to prevent opposing players from hurting key personnel. In the 1980s, Wayne Gretzky skated in the shadow of the fearsome Marty McSorley. If an opposing player hit Gretzky too hard, McSorley took to the ice and sent a message. The message usually involved the dropping of the gloves and a short, but memorable, series of punches to the head. The enforcer is a necessary component to a winning hockey team.

Antitumor agents are the enforcers of any effective cancer treatment program. Unfortunately, many patients do not recover when they choose surgery, radiation, or chemotherapy as an antitumor agent. This is not because those therapies fail to destroy cancerous tumors. They do destroy tumors quite effectively in many cases. The problem is that they do nothing to help the body's immune system. In fact, these therapies depress the immune system, thereby making long-term recuperation very difficult.

This area of the Oasis of Hope's medical treatment program is much more effective for two reasons. First, the Oasis research team has introduced a number of antitumor agents that are just as effective, but that are natural and do not present negative side effects. Many patients who stopped responding to chemotherapy have responded to these natural cancer killers. Second, our program supports the use of antitumor agents in conjunction with the support of detoxification and immunotherapy. The benefit to the patient is that this comprehensive approach greatly minimizes the negative side affects associated with cancer treatment. In most cancer centers, patients suffer from the treatment, but at Oasis most patients feel quite well and maintain a positive attitude.

## Alteration of Lifestyle

While patients receive treatment at Oasis, we begin to educate them on how to live healthy lives when they return home and how to continue therapy. Oasis doctors and nurses work with patients and their loved ones to teach them how to effectively self-administer therapies. This is a very cost-effective way for patients to continue therapy for a prolonged period of time.

In my many years of experience at the Oasis of Hope Hospital, I have observed that the patients who get the best results are those who make a real commitment to the program, the ones who have the discipline and desire to adhere to the therapies prescribed. A tragic error that many patients make is to abandon therapy as soon as they start to feel better or when they experience remission. Those who continue therapy, adhere to the nutrition program, and come back for the follow-up program gain the best results.

This is why the hospital's administration developed a program for patients to come back every six months for a two-day follow-up visit with their doctors at no charge. The follow-up program lasts a full five years at no additional cost to the patient. At these follow-up visits all the doctors monitor the patient's progress and make any modifications to the home care therapy that will better meet the patient's healthcare needs. I believe that the periodic phone calls we make to the patients have been vital because people need the encouragement and need to know that their doctor really cares.

I encourage every patient to completely adhere to the therapies and embrace the lifestyle changes we recommend at Oasis. I believe that a patient's commitment to the therapy is the single most important factor that determines how effective treatment is. That is why this final component of the Oasis medical treatment program is just as vital as the others.

# CHAPTER FIVE

## Coming Into Focus

My wife is prone to exaggeration. I know this because of an experience I had early on in our marriage. I was downstairs in the kitchen rummaging around for something to snack on when I heard a blood-curdling scream coming from our bedroom. I rushed to the base of the stairs and called up, "What happened?"

"Get up here, there's a bug on the wall by the nightstand!" she said. I rolled my eyes and began the trek upstairs.

I remembered the countless times my brother and I had played with bugs as kids. We used to trap separate species in a jar and watch them battle. Wasp vs. Bumble Bee, Praying Mantis vs. June Bug, etc. "What kind of bug is it?" I hollered.

"It's a huge spider…practically the size of my hand!" she replied, as I reached the landing. Now I was worried. The thought of a tarantula nesting somewhere in my bedroom was not a pleasant one. First of all, they are a lot faster than people imagine. They also have teeth. I don't like bugs with teeth. Then there's the issue of how big of a mess they make when you smash them.

I walked down the hall and entered the bedroom. My wife was on the far side of the room penned in safely behind a barrier she had constructed with two chairs. If she could have moved the dresser, she would have used that, too. I slipped off my shoe and determined that it had the right amount of heft to do some serious damage. "Where is it?" I asked.

She pointed a trembling hand at the nightstand on the far side of the bed. "It crawled down the wall behind there," she indicated. I tip-toed around the edge of the bed, giving a wide berth to the bed skirt, just in case the spider heard me coming and decided to perform a flanking maneuver. Moving perhaps a millimeter a minute I peered down the backside of the nightstand.

"Do you see it?" my wife shrieked. I shook my head. There was nothing on the wall except a cricket the size of my thumbnail. "It's not there, now," I shrugged. My wife had slid out from behind her furniture fortress, walked over and looked over the nightstand.

"There it is!" she screamed, and ran out of the room. It took me a minute to realize that the tiny cricket resting along the baseboard was, in fact, the man-eating spider in my wife's imagination. I had no problem taking care of the situation.

What I learned from the experience is that perception is everything. My wife's experience with bugs was different from mine. It had led her to believe that bugs are big, bad, ugly, and hungry for blood. My experience had led me to understand that bugs are cool, unless they have teeth. Perception is everything.

It is the understanding of this simple truth that leads us to perform a series of diagnostic tests and conduct a thorough interview when patients come to the Oasis of Hope Hospital. A physician's diagnosis is often shaped by perception. Much like eyewitnesses at an accident scene give accounts of the incident that vary greatly, the professional perspective of a physician will skew a diagnosis.

First, we want to verify that the diagnosis given to the patient was correct. Believe it or not, we had to refuse to treat a couple of patients who were diagnosed with cancer because further tests revealed that they did not have the disease after all. More commonly, our diagnostic tests will uncover more predictable inaccuracies, such as the type of cancer identified and the extent of the cancer's progression.

Second, we want to measure the rate at which the cancer is progressing. Often, we compare test results over a period of time. The comparison helps us to determine the effectiveness of previous treatment. For example, say in May a patient's tumor is measured at three centimeters. If comparative study reveals that the same tumor measured one centimeter in April, we know that the cancer grew in the interim and did not respond to the previous treatment.

Third, we want to set our own benchmark, in order to determine the effectiveness of our own treatment programs. If we administer a therapy and then use a reference point established from a different center's test results in conjunction with our own lab work, the analysis is likely to be highly inaccurate. In fact, it is not uncommon for diagnostic testing to vary greatly from one place to the next because of differences in lab conditions, testing materials, and testing techniques. The practice of comparing results from a variety of laboratories can truly create a situation where apples are compared to oranges.

Finally, we want to interpret the results of the diagnostic tests from our perspective. The doctors at the Oasis of Hope do not view cancer as an insurmountable obstacle. Our success with the total care approach of treating body, mind, and spirit has shaped a much more hopeful perspective. Couple this with the success we have seen with alternative treatment methods and our perspective brightens further.

We are not governed by a rigid medical community that is unwilling to abandon inhumane and ineffective treatments. Other doctors are. We are not pressured by huge pharmaceutical corporations interested only in boosting profit margins. Other doctors are. We are not crippled by years of failure and ever-rising mortality rates. Other doctors are. It is no wonder many mainstream doctors issue hopeless diagnoses. Their experience has cast a shadow of hopelessness on their perspective.

Our experience is not the same. Our perspective is not the same. There is hope. There is a way. Let me tell you in the next chapter where that road to health begins.

# Chapter Six

## Natural Defense System

I grew up on National Geographic television specials. Weren't they just the best? I remember watching a series on the great savannahs of Africa. I still feel sorry for the poor little antelopes that met their demises as the cheetah, a fierce and skilled predator, would do what he was born to do. It is amazing how this lighting fast cat can have such patience. He would lie in wait just below the tall amber grass. He would watch in silence just waiting for the perfect opportunity. If one little antelope would fall behind, the cheetah would strike.

Cancer is an opportunistic disease. If the conditions are right, any cell in the entire body can mutate. Mutations occur within the DNA. Malignant cells develop on a daily basis but they are extinguished or reprogrammed back to being a normal cell by the body's natural defense system if all is well. In its pristine condition, the human body is a strong fortress designed to fend off a frightening number of attacks daily. Any physician who tells you that keeping your body's defenses in tip-top shape is not the highest priority should be stripped of a license to practice. Cancer is lying in wait for any type of breakdown of the body's defense systems. When given the opportunity, cell mutation will begin and malignant cells will begin to reproduce at an uncontrollable, unstoppable rate. That is what cancer is. It is always a result of genetic abnormalities that are inherited or provoked by negative stressors. Should we fear the possibility of DNA fragmentation and cell mutation? No. We should dedicate ourselves to maintaining the function of the immune system.

Let's take a closer look at how the immune system works to prevent the proliferation of mutated cells. The immune system is made up of organs and cells that form a team to protect the body from outside agents that could be harmful. Certain cells are able to distinguish between normal and abnormal cells. When an abnormal or foreign cell is detected, these cells will seek them out and destroy them. There are many different types of cells that make up the immune system including monocytes, macrophages and neutrophils. The specific cells that combat cancer are in the group called lymphocytes, which are one type of white blood cell including B cells, T cells and Natural Killer (NK) cells.

T cells will directly attach to and attack cancerous cells. They are able to reproduce themselves through cloning right at the site of the abnormal cell. They perform another important function. T cells sound the "battle cry" and call into action NK cells. The NK cells are little chemical factories that produce highly potent substances that will attach themselves and kill anything that is foreign to the body. When the T and NK cells complete the destruction of the cancer cells, macrophages and phagocytes will absorb the dead cells and take them for elimination. This is where it is important to make sure that the lymphatic system, the liver, kidney, lungs and bowels are functioning properly as well.

A properly functioning immune system is the best way to prevent cancer but it is necessary to prevent a recurrence of cancer after treatment. The problem with most conventional therapies, especially chemotherapy, is that it destroys the white blood cells. For long-term remission of cancer, an adequate white blood cell count is indispensable. I found that, if a person is taking chemotherapy, a natural substance called AHCC will protect the blood cell count. I will talk about AHCC in chapter eight.

Again, strengthening the body's natural defense mechanism is the highest priority in the battle against disease. Nothing should compromise that goal.

Cancer causes a systemic dysfunction. The tumors are merely symptoms of a much larger problem. I also believe that conventional medicine continues to fail in the battle against cancer, because it has not reached the understanding of how abnormal cells function. DNA research has still been unable to reveal this mystery. As long as doctors focus on the tumor as the point of origin, they will be limited to a "band-aid" approach to cancer treatment. They will continue to fail in their efforts to halt the advance of the disease. Doctors need to embrace a different perspective. They need to see the tumor as the red flag. They need to determine what the body needs to restore its natural defenses and reprogram mutated cells.

Let's take a moment to organize the concepts I am presenting here. The failing of most treatments today is that they only attack the tumors. But tumors are the symptom of cancer. There is no doubt that an effective program should try to reverse or halt growth of tumors but that will not be sufficient to avoid a relapse. Immune function must be addressed as well because a depressed immune system leaves the door wide open for cancer to come back with a vengeance. But this is still not enough. Immune dysfunction provides cancer the opportunity needed to develop but it is not the cause of cancer.

It is important to detect what is stressing the body and its immune system. These stressors number in the tens of thousands so it may be impossible to identify the cause of a patient's cancer. There must be thousands of unknown causes to complicate things further. What we know is that negative stressors generate damaging oxygen free radicals that destabilize normal cells. A patient and physician must put on their detective caps to at least identify glaring stressors that could be eliminated from the patient's lifestyle. Most of the time, patients have to figure these things out because it takes a lot of time and thought and the time a patient spends with a doctor is usually insufficient. I would like to present a list of stressors that are related to cancer. This is just to help you get started in thinking about the concept. It is not comprehensive by any means. For example, there are over 30,000 carcinogens identified just in the chemical industry. It would not be possible to provide a complete list. But consider the following to motivate you to look for ways to improve your lifestyle and surroundings.

## I. DIET AND NUTRITIONAL FACTORS
(represents 60% and 40% of all cancers in women
and men, respectively).
- Fat intake
- High intake of animal protein
- Smoked foods
- Salt-cured foods
- Fried, broiled or barbecued meat, chicken or fish
- Pesticides found in food
- Food additives
- Alcohol
- High intake of caffeine

## II. SMOKING
(It is the single major cause of cancer death
accounting for 30% of all deaths)

## III. ENVIRONMENTAL TOXICITY
- PCBs
- Garden pesticides
- Herbicides
- Contaminated soil, water and air
- Asbestos
- Indoor pollution (fumes and vapors produced by cleaning products, paints, hobby supplies, radon, among others)
- Chlorinated drinking water

## IV. ENVIRONMENTAL RADIATION
- Electromagnetic fields
- Nuclear energy
- UV Radiation (solar radiation)

## V. Stress and Psychological Factors
- Depression
- Stress

## VI. Genetics
- BRCA1
- BRCA2

## VII. Viruses
- Hepatitis B virus
- Herpes simplex 2
- CMV (Cytomegalovirus)

As I said, the list could be endless. Considering the fact that we are in daily contact with tens of thousands of cancer-causing agents, it is a miracle that everyone doesn't get cancer. When you consider all of the variables involved in what causes cancer, the importance of a properly functioning immune system, and actually trying to reverse cancer, it becomes very apparent that a cure-all magic bullet really doesn't exist. It is only realistic to think that we can engage a patient into a process to slowly undue cancer.

# CHAPTER SEVEN

## *Cleaning House*

One of my favorite things to do in the afternoon is to catch the show "Iron Chef" on the Food Network. If you've never seen it, you don't know what you're missing. The show is a cross between Home Run Derby, the WWF, and figure skating. Iron Chef pits two world-renowned chefs against each other in head-to-head competition, much like Home Run Derby used to pit two of baseball's biggest sluggers against each other. The chef's engage in a good deal of trash talking before, during, and after the competition, much like the steroid-injected wrestlers of the WWF. The artistic abilities of the two chefs are evaluated by a panel of judges, much like a figure skating competition. What a concept!

The thing that impresses me most about the chefs featured on the show is how clean they keep the workspace, even in the heat of battle. I can totally identify with that mind set. I won't even think about starting to cook until all dirty dishes from previous meals are loaded into the dishwasher and the food prep area is spotless. I can't think clearly if I have to work around stacks of dirty plates and utensils. When the workspace is clean and organized, I'm at my absolute best.

The same can be said about the body. The body possesses amazing self-healing mechanisms, but an imbalanced and unclean working environment often hampers these talents. As we live our lives, our bodies absorb an unbelievable number of environmental and food-borne toxins. The body works hard to eliminate these toxins and keep the internal workspace pure and clean. Unfortunately, our dietary and lifestyle choices often make it impossible for the body to keep up with the flood of incoming toxins. Thus, the body's internal environment suffers a build-up of these substances and its ability to heal itself is compromised. Therefore, one of the first steps in a comprehensive cancer treatment program is to clean up the internal workspace.

At the Oasis of Hope we offer Chelation therapy to all our patients, using a synthetic aminoacid known as ethylene diamine tetraacetic acid (EDTA), silymarin, and vitamin C. We incorporate foods that have powerful detoxification properties into the hospital diet. Finally, we recommend that all of our patients consult a doctor who practices biological dentistry.

The word *chelation* comes from the Greek root *chele* meaning "to bind." The concept is relatively simple. Chelation therapy involves the introduction of a substance into the body that will bind to harmful substances and pull them out of the body. It is an extremely safe and effective method of ridding the body of toxic substances.

EDTA is a synthetic amino acid that is featured in Chelation therapy. Our bodies often store a host of toxic metals, such as lead, iron, copper, cadmium, aluminum, and calcium. Needless to say, the presence of these substances dirties the internal workspace and hampers the body's ability to heal itself. When EDTA is administered intravenously, it binds to these toxic metals in the blood.[1] This makes it easier for the body to flush these harmful substances through the kidneys.

Chelation therapy with EDTA was first used in the United States in 1950 to treat the lead poisoning suffered by workers in a Michigan battery factory.[2] The treatment was highly successful, because EDTA is especially equipped to remove iron and copper, which are powerful catalysts of lipid peroxidation and free radical formation. Chelation therapy is an effective tool in the effort to detoxify the body and minimize the damages of degenerative diseases.[3]

Another detoxification agent used in Chelation therapy is silymarin, a substance found in the seeds of a common herb known as milk thistle. Silymarin is actually a collection of disease-fighting substances called polyphenolic flavonoids.[4] Milk thistle has been used medicinally for more than 2000 years, especially as a liver protector.

Silymarin has been used clinically to treat a variety of conditions. These include toxic hepatitis, viral hepatitis, cirrhosis of the liver, ischaemic injury, and radiation toxicity. Doctors marvel at the anti-oxidative, anti-lipid-peroxidative, anti-fibrotic, anti-inflammatory, immunomodulating, and liver regenerating effects of silymarin.[5] Let me explain two of these in detail.

Several studies have shown that silymarin is an amazingly strong antioxidant. It is capable of destroying both free radicals and reactive oxygen species, substances that cause significant damage to cells. Doing so decreases the damage these substances cause cells. Healthier cells are more capable of defending themselves against these substances. Thus, the use of silymarin has a double effect. The first effect is the destruction of harmful substances, resulting in healthier cells. The second effect is the enhancement of cellular defense machinery, resulting in the destruction of even more harmful substances.[6] In addition, it is this antioxidant property that protects the liver, pancreas, kidney, red cells, and platelets from the toxic effects of alcohol, carbon tetrachloride, cold ischemia, industrial toxins, and drug toxins.[7]

Silymarin also helps restructure liver cells to prevent toxins from penetrating the organ and stimulates the regenerative ability of the liver by helping form new cells.[8] The liver is one of the most powerful cleaning tools the body possesses. The healthier the liver is, the more effectively the body can rid itself of toxins. Researchers found that silymarin increases the content of liver glutathione, a potent antioxidant that helps regulate the removal of toxins from liver cells.[9] Glutathione is considered the most important agent the body has to battle chemically-induced toxicity.

Moreover, silymarin is largely free of adverse effects, even at large doses. It is one of the safest and most effective tools we can use to clean up the internal environment and empower the body to heal itself. A treatment program that does not offer silymarin deprives patients of a powerful weapon against disease.

Another chelating agent we use in our therapy is vitamin C. For years, doctors have known that vitamin C protects the body against a variety of pollutants.[10] As a detoxification agent, vitamin C combines with certain toxins in the body and destroys them.[11] What research tells us is that vitamin C is especially good at eliminating toxins that originate from airborne sources, like cigarette smoke. Some laboratory experiments showed that the protein and lipid damage caused by cigarette smoke is reversed when the subject eliminates exposure and undergoes vitamin C therapy.[12]

Other studies indicate that vitamin C can protect the body against the tissue-damaging effect of some toxic chemicals and heavy metals. One study compared the chelating properties of vitamin C to EDTA and found them to have equivalent activity with respect to lead.[13] The combined use of EDTA, silymarin, and vitamin C in chelation therapy results in a gentle but thorough detoxification of the body's internal workspace. Remember, cleaning the workspace allows the body to operate at maximum capacity. Any treatment program that does not attempt to equip the body to combat disease, is deficient in its approach.

Ever seen those commercials for high-grade gasoline? Every company wants to impress upon you the importance of putting the right kind of fuel in your car. Well, food is fuel for the body. If we desire to detoxify the body in order to fight disease, we must put the right kind of fuel in it. There are many foods that are abundant sources of antioxidants and other detoxification agents. At the Oasis of Hope, we are intentional about incorporating those foods into the hospital diet we offer every patient. I will talk about some of those whole foods and natural substances in the next chapter.

As I mentioned earlier, we are exposed to a host of toxins every day in the air we breathe, the foods we eat, and the water we drink. However, there are some sources of toxic substances of which most people are woefully unaware. Consider your teeth, for example. Do you have any fillings, bridges, or partials? Have you ever had a root canal performed?

Few cancer specialists have ever considered having a patient's mouth examined. Oncologists need to be aware of the connection between cancer and the mercury in tooth fillings, as well as other materials used in dentistry that are carcinogenic. Believe it or not, most oncologists today don't care about the dental work their patients have had and most dentists continue to use toxic materials for fillings, bridges, and partials.

Dr. Hal Huggins, a world-renowned dentist and immunologist, has helped me to understand the importance of biological dentistry. It is not simply the practice of removing toxic fillings. The whole practice also involves finding non-toxic materials that are compatible with each patient. Another doctor named Dr. Thomas Levy developed effective lab tests to determine what materials are or are not compatible for a patient.

At Oasis, we work with Dr. Ezekiel Lagos, a dentist that has studied with Dr. Huggins and Dr. Levy. Dr. Lagos has practiced biological dentistry for many years. His programs are comprehensive and designed to remove the toxic dental work that can compromise the body's immune system. One of many services he provides is the removal of amalgams, which are fillings that use mercury in the alloy.

His protocol is amazingly thorough. First, he performs a serum compatibility test of dental materials to determine which dental materials are most compatible with the patient's immune system. Next, he prescribes vitamin C tablets, minerals, and digestive enzymes a few weeks prior to the total dental revision (TDR) procedure to protect the body from the toxins present in the fillings.

Then, the TDR procedure is performed, which includes the removal of fillings in the proper sequence, using a rubber dam. All biologically incompatible fillings are removed and replaced with the most biocompatible replacement materials. All identifiable sources of dental infection are removed, including all cavities and implants.

The precautions he exercises are commendable. Extra water and negative ion generators are used during treatment to reduce the amount of mercury vapor in the office environment. Intravenous vitamin C is administered before, during, and after the TDR procedure. This helps neutralize any toxins that reach the blood and tissues.

After the procedure is complete, Dr. Lagos takes additional measures to care for the patient. He administers Protamina Zinc Insulin (PZI) to increase circulation and stimulate formation of new blood vessels. This helps to speed the healing process. Because healing progresses faster without pain medication, strong negative pole magnets are applied to all operative sites after the dental work and acupressure is performed at the conclusion of dental treatment. This completely eliminates the need for pain medications in many patients.

Dr. Lagos educates his patients, explaining which measures will most effectively treat and possibly reverse any periodontal disease that may be present. Toxic dental work can have such a devastating impact on the immune system that you should not put off seeing a good biological dentist.

When the toxins present in the body are removed and the internal environment is thoroughly cleaned, the body is prepared to battle disease. To enter into battle weak and ill-prepared is foolish. This is why a solid detoxification program is an integral part of a comprehensive cancer treatment program.

# CHAPTER EIGHT

## *Nature's Pharmacy*

I don't know if you know anything about the game of softball, or not, but I've learned that having the proper equipment is very important. I remember sitting in the stands at a friend's game absolutely dumbfounded at the ability of the players to hit the ball great distances. I have played before and I can hit the ball a long way, but not every time. These players were driving every ball deep into the outfield it seemed. They weren't all mammoth-sized freaks of nature, either. I just about died when their tiny shortstop, who couldn't have been much bigger than a three-drawer filing cabinet, stepped up and sent the ball screaming over the left field fence. Later, I learned their secret.

You see, not all softball bats are alike. There are softball bats and then there are *softball bats*. The bats these guys were using were double-walled bats manufactured by the DiMarini company. These bats run upwards of three-hundred dollars. What they do is provide a little extra boost to your swing and add about fifty to sixty feet to your hit. The right equipment makes a noticeable difference in a team's ability to hit the ball deep.

The same is true of the body's ability to ward off degenerative diseases like cancer. Given the right equipment, the body is remarkably adept at healing itself. Sadly, we often deprive our bodies of the very tools it needs to do this job effectively. If these tools were hard to come by, we might have an excuse, but the reality is that they are readily available.

Hippocrates, the father of medicine, said, "Let your food be your medicine and your medicine be your food." The human body needs the right equipment to fight off disease and maintain optimal health. Hippocrates knew that many of the tools our bodies need to heal are found in the natural world. Tools like phytochemicals, proteins, enzymes, vitamins, and minerals do not need to be manufactured in the laboratories of some pharmaceutical company. The foundational elements of the Oasis of Hope's drive to bolster the body's immune system are whole foods and totally natural substances.

Whole foods are foods that have not been processed, manipulated, or manufactured by men. Instead, they exist in the same state that God designed in the Garden of Eden. I firmly believe that the foods and food extracts we prescribe are as important, if not more important, than the pharmaceuticals we prescribe. The right foods alone can effectively combat some cancers.

We know that free radical activity is at the root of cancer. We know that a host of things can increase the presence of free radicals in the body, from smoking cigarettes to eating processed foods. We know that free radicals can damage DNA cells and the gene expression process. When these damaged cells reproduce, the result is often cancer and tumor development. Therefore, anything that can significantly inhibit tumor growth, improve gene expression, or scavenge free radicals is a tool the body needs to fight off cancer. There are so many of these natural cancer killers that I could write a whole book about them. Here are a few of the more important ones that we use and recommend at Oasis.

*Aged Garlic Extract*

Garlic and aged garlic extract is an integral part of the effort to equip the body to ward off disease. Garlic is one of the most studied whole foods. The Wakunaga Company, producers of Kyolic Aged Garlic Extract, is committed to the study of the health benefits associated with their product. I began using Kyolic Aged Garlic Extract as a natural antibiotic to treat ear infections. It worked wonders with my kids. It earned a permanent spot in my medicine bag when I discovered its effectiveness as an antistress and antifatigue agent. When recent research demonstrated the role garlic plays in the health of the heart, a thought occurred to me.

I wondered, "Could garlic present similar benefits to cancer patients and people wishing to avoid the disease?" I began to review the medical literature. I was thrilled to find that Aged Garlic Extract constituents have been shown to be effective in inhibiting the growth and development of prostate cancer cells,[1] melanoma cells[2] and neuroblastoma cells.[3] In addition, these constituents slow the growth and development of carcinogen-induced tumors of the bladder,[4] breast,[5] colon,[6] esophagus,[7] stomach,[8] and lung.[9]

I was impressed with the extensive nature of these clinical studies. Li G and collaborators[10] found that two elements in aged garlic extract, called S-ally cysteine (SAC) and S-allyl mercaptocysteine, inhibit the growth and proliferation of breast cancer cells. Not only do they slow the development of breast cancer cells, but they also equip surrounding cells with tools they desperately need, like gluthathione-S-transferase and peroxidase. These elements are critical agents in cell detoxification and gene expression. In other words, these elements help cells get rid of the toxins that damage their ability to reproduce properly. Remember, when the gene expression process is compromised, the result is often a cancerous cell.

Much of garlic's activity derives from aliin and allicin or its immediate byproducts as S-allyl cysteine and S-allyl-mercaptocysteine found in aged garlic extracts.[11] Also garlic contains the minerals selenium and tellurium.

Among other aged garlic's extract attributes are its anti-infection,[12] antiaging,[13] cardioprotective,[14] and immune enhancement[15] properties.

Aged garlic extract has the ability to prolong life span, improve learning and spatial memory,[16] prevent the decrease in brain weight and the atrophic changes in frontal brain[17] in senescence-accelerated mouse. These results suggest that Aged Garlic Extract might be useful for treating physiological aging and age-related memory disorders in humans.

I am not claiming that garlic can cure cancer but I am firmly stating that the constituents in aged garlic extract are important in combating carcinogens within the body. Thank God for garlic!

## Tomatoes

The tomato is another excellent source of disease-fighting equipment. The tomato is one of the richest sources of a powerful antioxidant called *lycopene*. Antioxidants are substances that scavenge free radicals. Remember, free radicals can damage cells and the gene expression process. Several epidemiological studies show that the regular intake of tomatoes and tomato products is associated with a lower risk of several cancers.[18] A case-control study of an elderly population linked the consistent intake of tomato lycopene to protective effects against digestive tract cancers and a 50 percent reduction in death from cancer.[19]

Giovannucci[20] recently reviewed seventy-two epidemiological studies. These included ecological, case-control, dietary, and blood-specimen-based investigations. All the studies examined the effect of tomato lycopene on cancer. In the majority of these studies there was an inverse association between tomato intake and the risk of several types of cancer. In other words, the more tomatoes a person ate, the lower their risk of getting cancer was.

What is important is that in thirty-five of these studies, the inverse associations were statistically significant. The evidence for benefit was strongest for cancers of the prostate, lung, and stomach. Data also suggested benefit for cancers of the pancreas, colon, rectum, esophagus, oral cavity, breast, and cervix. None of the studies showed adverse effects of high tomato intake.

Prostate cancer is the most common cancer and second leading cause of cancer mortality in men in the United States.[21] Recent studies have suggested a potential benefit of tomato lycopene against the risk of prostate cancer, particularly the more lethal forms of this cancer.[22] An 83 percent reduction of prostate cancer risk was observed in individuals with the highest plasma concentration of lyco-pene, compared to individuals with the lowest concentration.[23]

I have been working very closely with a company named Wil-son-Batiz to develop the most natural, pesticide-free tomatoes with very high concentrations of lycopene. These tomatoes are being sent to an FDA approved lab in the USA to verify the high content of lycopene. Why do I mention this? Not only will these tomatoes be used as a part of the Oasis of Hope treatment program but they will soon be available in all major grocery stores. I applaud Wilson-Batiz for producing biologically functional foods without the use of chemi-cals and introducing them to the general public.

## Melatonin

Another one of nature's wonders is a substance called melatonin. This neuro-hormone is synthesized and secreted at night by the pi-neal gland, which is located in the brain.[24] Studies have found that melatonin is a highly effective antitumor agent. Melatonin does a num-ber of important things. It inhibits the proliferation of cancer cells, stimulates mechanisms that fight cancer, encourages proper gene ex-pression, and scavenges free radicals.[25]

Several clinical studies provide strong evidence suggesting me-latonin can inhibit cancer cell growth.[26] In one clinical study, melato-nin was administered to 1,440 patients with "untreatable" tumors.[27] In another study, melatonin was given to 200 patients with chemo-therapy–resistant tumors.[28] In both studies, the frequency of cachexia,[29] asthenia,[30] thrombocytopenia,[31] and lymphocytopenia[32] was significantly lower for patients treated with melatonin than the control group. Moreover, the percentage of patients with disease stabilization was significantly higher for patients treated with melato-nin than in the control group.[33] In other words, the melatonin ap-peared to slow or halt the development of existing tumors.

Other studies indicate that melatonin stimulates some of the mechanisms in the body that combat cancer. For example, studies show that melatonin amplifies the antitumoral activity of interleukin–2.[34] Scientists have also determined that a reduction in melatonin concentration can cause deficiency in immune function. One result of this is a reduction in tumor surveillance, the body's ability to recognize and combat tumor growth. The immune surveillance system plays a critical role in prevention of cancer by recognizing the formation of abnormal cells. T-cells in particular are valuable for their ability to distinguish mutated cells from normal cells. Yet, when the immune system is suppressed, the mutated carcinoma cells are not recognized by the immune surveillance system and the cells grow uncontrollably and become cancerous. When the body gets enough melatonin, the tumor surveillance system functions properly.

In order for cells to reproduce properly they have to be able to accurately receive genetic instructions. Studies show that melatonin increases the gap-junction-intercellular communication.[35] Most cancer cells have some dysfunction in gap-junction-intercellular communication. In addition, many tumor-promoting chemicals cause this dysfunction in intercellular communication, whereas chemicals like melatonin improve intercellular communication.[36] The better the communication, the less likely a cell is to produce cancer.

Finally, melatonin is one of the most powerful antioxidants found in nature. Research shows that it protects DNA, cell membranes, lipids, and proteins from free-radical damage.[37] An important quality of melatonin is its ability to enter all cells of the body and every subcellular compartment.[38] This means that melatonin can enter a cell's nucleus and scavenge the free radicals responsible for DNA damage.[39] Since the radical-scavenging function of melatonin is dose-dependent, a decreased melatonin concentration is directly connected with a diminished protection of DNA, leading to a higher risk of cancer.[40] Melatonin is a highly effective scavenger of the hydroxyl free radicals, which is considered the most damaging of all the free radicals.[41] For all of these reasons, the administration of melatonin is a part of the Oasis program. We believe it is a tool the body can use to ward off disease.

*AHCC*

Another way to bolster the immune system is with the use of Active Hexose Correlated Compound (AHCC), an extract obtained from several kinds of mushroom. Mushroom extracts are known to have immuno-modulating and antitumor effects.[42] AHCC is very effective in strengthening and optimizing the capacity of the immune system. The Oasis clinical research organization conducted a study comparing patients taking chemotherapy combined with AHCC and another group taking chemotherapy alone. One of the nasty side effects of chemotherapy is that it can severely depress the immune system. We found that AHCC truly protected the immune system from the depressing effects of chemotherapy. AHCC can reduce the side effects of radiotherapy, as well. AHCC also improves the patients' quality of life by reducing nausea, increasing appetite, and decreasing anxiety. Furthermore, there are no side effects to taking AHCC as an immune-enhancing supplement.

Like melatonin, AHCC also stimulates the immune surveillance system. Cancer cells release several kinds of immune suppressive factors, which inhibit the body's ability to combat the disease. When the immune system is suppressed, a chain reaction of sorts occurs which results in the inhibition of the antitumor effects which should come naturally to the body. The anticancer immune response fails when the production of killer cells fails. Thus, reversing and restoring the suppressed immune system is a very important part of cancer treatment.[43]

AHCC restores and reverses a depressed immune system by inhibiting the immune suppressive factors produced by the cancer cells, increasing production of the cells that attack cancer, and stimulating the activity of the killer cells in particular.[44] For this reason, AHCC is an important part of the well-rounded Oasis treatment program.

*Coenzyme Q10*

Another powerful agent is CoQ10, or Coenzyme Q10. This is a naturally occurring, fat-soluble substance that possesses vitamin-like properties. It is an essential component of the energy production process within our cells. While it is true that CoQ10 occurs naturally within the body, the levels of the substance decline as we age.[45] If a person has an addiction to cigarettes, high cholesterol, or heart disease these decreases can be significant.[46] There is clinical evidence linking cancer and immune system dysfunction to lowered levels of CoQ10.[47] What does this substance do that is so important?

It acts as an amazingly effective antioxidant by scavenging free radicals.[48] This means that CoQ10 defends against the onset of cancer and destroys existing cancer. One study[49] tracked patients with a variety of cancers. The study showed that 60 percent became free of the cancer during therapy with CoQ10.[50] Another report[51] noted partial remission of breast cancer in over 10 percent of the "high-risk" patients studied. These patients were treated with CoQ10. The same study also reported that the metastases of the cancer ceased during CoQ10 treatment.[52] Both the regression of the primary tumor and the end of metastases in these cases are understood to be the result of the stimulating activity of CoQ10 on the immune system.[53] Doctors would be foolish not to equip patients with this powerful, disease-fighting weapon.

## Olive Oil

Yet another functional food is olive oil, the principal source of fat in the Mediterranean diet. Olive oil has been associated with health benefits that include prevention of several varieties of cancers, and the bolstering of the immune system.[54] Olive oil contains components that contribute to its overall therapeutic characteristics. Extra-virgin olive oil contains a considerable amount of phenolic compounds such as tyrosol and oleuropein, which exhibit antioxidant effects.[55] Specifically, these compounds are excellent scavengers of free radicals.[56] Recent studies showed that phenolic compounds in olive oil help to suppress carcinogenesis.[57] It is so easy to incorporate things like olive oil into diet. We all should do it!

## Omega-3 Fatty Acids

The omega-3 fatty acids are not only essential nutrients, but are also fantastic disease fighters. Several thousand scientific publications testify to the widespread agreement among medical professionals regarding the benefits of omega-3 fatty acids. For years, doctors have recognized the benefits of the Mediterranean diet, a diet rich in omega-3 fatty acids. Studies show that individuals who get a sufficient amount of these fatty acids in their diet experience a significantly lower risk of cancer mortality.[58]

Some of the best sources of these acids are fish, plants, and oils. Fish are high in the omega-3 acids known as alpha-linolenic acid (ALA), eicosapentaenoic acid (EPA) and decosahexaenoic acid (DHA). Plants and oils contain the acid known as ALA. Of the plant sources; nuts, seeds, and soybeans are relatively high in ALA content.[59] The contents of ALA in soybean and canola oil is approximately 7.8 percent and 9.2 percent, respectively. Flaxseed oil is a particularly rich source of n-3 fatty acids mainly ALA with an average content ranged from 57-69 percent although it is not a commonly used food oil.[60] Table 2 (see page73) illustrates the AHA content of a variety of sources.

## Silymarin

Silymarin is a polyphenolic disease fighting agent derived from milk thistle.[61] Several studies have shown that silymarin is a very strong antioxidant, capable of scavenging both free radicals and reactive oxygen species, which results in a boost to cellular defense mechanisms.[62] For the last nine years, scientific researches have been studying the cancer chemopreventative and anticarcinogenic effects of silymarin. These studies have shown that silymarin affords exceptional protection against cancers of the skin, prostate, breast, lung, colon, and bladder.[63]

Not only does silymarin protect against the onset of cancer, but it can significantly inhibit the growth of existing cancer, as well. Two new studies show this inhibitory effect.[64] Researchers from these studies conclude that silymarin can be an effective agent for both prevention and intervention. So, how does it work?

One of the marks of cancer cells is the reckless abandon with which they reproduce. Silymarin inhibits this cell proliferation and alters the cell cycle progression in various types of cancer.[65] When this happens, the cancer cells begin to suffer substantial apoptotic death, or programmed death.[66] The interruption to the cell cycle helps the body to differentiate between healthy cells and cancer cells, thus enabling the body's immune system to target the cancer more effectively.[67] Currently the Oasis scientists and chemists are developing a pharmaceutical grade silymarin solution that can be administered through injection. I have high hopes that it will prove to be a convenient and powerful antitumor agent. Stay tuned!

The study of functional, whole foods and natural, disease-fighting substances is just beginning. The modern medical community has barely opened the door of nature's medicine chest. I encourage you to get online and learn as much as you can about these things and put them to work for your health.

TABLE 2: TERRESTRIAL PLANT SOURCES OF ALPHA-LINOLENIC
ACID (ALA;18:3N-3) *

| Source (100g edible portion, raw) | Alpha-linolenic acid (g) (ALA) |
|---|---|
| *Nuts and seeds* | |
| Almonds | 0.4 |
| Flaxseed | 22.8 |
| Mixed nuts | 0.2 |
| Peanuts | 0.003 |
| Pecans | 0.7 |
| Soybean kennels | 1.5 |
| Walnuts, black | 3.3 |
| Walnuts, English and Persian | 6.8 |
| *Vegetables and legumes* | |
| Beans, navy and pinto, sprouted (cooked) | 0.3 |
| Broccoli (raw) | 0.1 |
| Cauliflower | 0.1 |
| Lentils (dry) | 0.1 |
| Lima beans (dry) | 0.2 |
| Peas, garden (dry) | 0.2 |
| Radish seeds, sprouted (raw) | 0.7 |
| Soybeans, green (raw) | 3.2 |
| Soybeans (dry) | 1.6 |
| Spinach (raw) | 0.1 |
| *Grains* | |
| Barley, bran | 0.3 |
| Corn, germ | 0.3 |
| Oats, germ | 1.4 |
| Rice, bran | 0.2 |
| Wheat, bran | 0.2 |
| Wheat, germ | 0.7 |
| *Fruit* | |
| Avocados (raw) | 0.1 |
| Raspberries (raw) | 0.1 |
| Strawberries (raw) | 0.1 |

* Data from Kris-Etherton PM, Taylor DS, Yu-Poth S et al. Polyunsaturated fatty acids in the food chain in the United States. Am J Clin Nutr 2000; 71 (Suppl):179S-188S.

# CHAPTER NINE

## *A Combined Effort*

One of my favorite board games ever is Risk. The object of the game is to conquer the world. You place your armies strategically around the board trying to capture territories held by opposing players, all the while seeking to protect those that you already possess. On the surface, it is a fascinating game of strategy, timing, and quick thinking. Beneath the surface, however, is an even more fascinating game of alliances.

Much like the game of Monopoly, the game of Risk has a reputation for dragging on for days. This is due to the unseen aspect of the game I mentioned. As a player, I noticed that whenever an opponent began to gain momentum, gobbling up surrounding territories, an unspoken alliance was formed between the other players in an attempt to restore balance to the board. If your attempt to win was too heavy-handed, you were sure to face the combined efforts of the rest of the players. Needless to say, heavy-handed attempts to rule the world rarely won the game. Just ask Hitler.

Cancer is heavy-handed. There is nothing subtle at all about the presence of a malignant tumor in your kidney or lung. Cancer makes no attempt to veil its threat. It is a disease that gathers momentum quickly and attacks with frightening ferocity. Only a concerted and combined effort can repel such an attack. This is the principle behind the Metabolic Therapy my father pioneered.

My father believed that to defeat cancer, it was necessary to attack it from every possible angle. He understood the importance of both direct and indirect approaches. The foundation of the Metabolic Therapy is its multi-faceted approach. Yes, we do attack the tumor, but we also stimulate the immune system and address causal factors. Our total care approach requires the patient's participation. Cancer treatment is not a spectator's sport. The patient must be prepared for the fight. We go through a process of structuring a patient for success by providing the necessary resources to face the threat at the physical, emotional, and spiritual levels. There is no question that the alliance between body, mind, and spirit can even the playing field against cancer. In chapters that follow, I will take you through our newest therapies as well as mind/spirit medicine but let me begin with the foundational program my father designed to dismantle cancer's strongholds. In this chapter, I will share how we can sensitize cancer to treatment, attack the tumor, cut off its supply lines, and take out cancer's transportation system.

Let´s start with sensitizing the tumor. Did you know that cancer defends itself against attacks? Tumors can become resistant to chemotherapy, radiation or whatever else you throw at it. It would make sense that if you could dismantle cancer's defenses, you could then take it out, right? What are the ways that cancer defends itself? One way is that tumors encapsulate themselves with blood vessels that are so restricted that antitumor agents can't get through. Another way is that tumors amass high concentrations of a substance called *glutathione*. Glutathione is the element that makes tumors resistant to treatment. Is there a way to lower the levels of glutathione in tumors so that they would become sensitized to anticancer treatments? The answer is yes. For glutathione to be produced in the cells, it needs another substance called *cysteine*. Please continue with me on this trail that it took many years to identify by top researchers. Is there a way to lower the level of cysteine? Yes. Cyanide will deplete the supply of cysteine. But, isn't cyanide a poison? Cyanide is toxic to our body but it will not make us sick in very low doses derived from a whole food source. You eat cyanide-rich food everyday if you eat apricots, pineapples, apples, or any of the other thousand cyanide-toting foods found in nature. The cyanide in these

76

foods is present in a nutrient called *amygdalin*. Amygdalin can release cyanide within malignant cells, depleting the supply of cysteine. As a result, the intracellular concentration of glutathione is diminished. This will sensitize the tumors to antitumor treatments including chemotherapy, Ozone therapy, and UV light.

We also use amygdalin to attack the tumor. The cyanide released by amygdalin is one of the best killers of malignant cells as well. Amygdalin has a double punch. It lowers cancers resistance to treatment and it releases cyanide to kill cancer cells directly. If you wish to read the technical explanation of how these two functions of amygdalin occur, please refer to appendices I and II at the end of the book.

If amygdalin can be so helpful, why aren't more cancer treatment centers using it? The first argument is that it can be toxic because it contains cyanide. The second argument is that it doesn't work.

Let's talk about amygdalin's toxicity first. We have used amygdalin with tens of thousands of patients since the early 1960s. You might say that we know a thing or two about amygdalin which is also known as *laetrile* and *vitamin B17*. The cyanide released by amygdalin does not reach toxic levels that can harm or even discomfort patients. But don't accept my word as the only proof. A famous researcher named June de Spain conducted a laetrile toxicity study that was published in *The Little Cyanide Cookbook* (Am. Media). She took three groups of rats. Group one was fed white bread. Group two was fed whole wheat bread. Group three was fed laetrile. After three months, 75 percent of rats that were eating white bread were dead. The white bread survivors were at death's door. The rats that were eating whole wheat bread were in good shape. The rats who were eating laetrile were all alive and in the best condition of the three groups. The conclusion of this FDA sponsored trial was that, "white bread is 70 times more toxic than laetrile." No, laetrile/amygdalin presents no risk of toxicity.

What about the argument that laetrile is not effective? We have conducted several prospective clinical trials that demonstrated that amygdalin is quite effective in the combined treatment of the most common and deadly cancers including inoperable lung cancer, advanced prostate cancer, stage IV breast cancer, and colon cancer with liver metastasis.[1] We submitted these studies to several medical journals but they were rejected. Some editors cited that our studies did not have control groups. But it is scientifically valid to conduct a study and compare results with similar studies published in medical journals. That is what we did but we were still denied publication. Other editors stated that our study was not designed properly and that the conclusion was not definitive. Others were quite candid. They rejected the studies because the use of amygdalin was too controversial. I think the third group was honest and I appreciated getting a straight answer from them.

The only study ever published on the use of laetrile in cancer patients was sponsored by the National Cancer Institute and conducted at the Mayo Clinic and three other prominent oncological centers in the USA. The results were published in *The New England Journal of Medicine* (*NEJM*) in 1982.

In this article "A clinical trial of amygdalin (laetrile) in the treatment of human cancer,"[2] Dr. Moertel, the head researcher, reported that of the 178 patients that were accepted in the study "not one patient was cured or even stabilized" by laetrile. Furthermore he said that "several patients experienced symptoms of cyanide toxicity" and that "blood levels of cyanide approaching the lethal range" were reported. "Laetrile has had its day in court…" says Moertel and ends authoritatively, "The evidence, beyond reasonable doubt, is that it [laetrile] doesn't benefit patients with advanced cancer, and there is no reason to believe that it would be any more effective in the earlier stages of the disease."

I was astonished at the finality of the verdict, but what disappointed me the most was the editorial bias of the *NEJM*. Why did the NCI and the Mayo Clinic bypass all scientific protocol? This study had no control group. It was terribly designed and not one of the researchers had any experience with laetrile. The *NEJM*, in normal conditions, will not publish studies that are not peer reviewed by experts on the subject. There are very few laetrile experts. I know all of them personally and the researchers consulted not one of us.

Years later, after a presentation at an oncology congress of our results in advanced breast cancer with amygdalin, a colleague angrily confronted me using the microphone placed in the center isle for questions. He was infuriated because I continued to use amygdalin in spite of the fact that Dr. Moertel, had *proven*, beyond reasonable doubt, that amygdalin was dangerous and ineffective. The scene was surreal; the room was filled to capacity, and, if a tongue depressor had fallen from a doctor's gown, all of us would have heard it. His forehead, which reached almost to the back of his head due to an almost complete male-pattern-baldness, was bright red, his jugulars were ingurgitated, and I didn't know if I wanted to run scared or laugh. But every one was waiting for my rebuttal.

Obviously he did not believe the results I had just presented which, by the way, were quite impressive. I took a deep breath and calmly asked, would you stop using Taxol (a chemotherapeutic agent used commonly in breast cancer) if I showed you *one* article that said it was not effective for the treatment of breast cancer? He just turned around and left. I assumed his jugulars were still ingurgitated because his baldhead turned even redder. There were no more questions because everyone in the room knew that there are dozens of studies showing the inefficacy and high toxicity of Taxol in the treatment of breast cancer, yet most oncologists continue to prescribe it.

Because of one study, amygdalin has been written off. Our positive experience with amygdalin obliges us to continue offering it to patients. I believe that it is irresponsible to state that amygdalin is a cancer cure. It should be looked at as a therapy that can be combined with conventional treatments or other antitumor agents. This is the appropriate future of amygdalin. At Oasis, we do not use amygdalin as a stand-alone drug. We capitalize on its ability to make tumors more susceptible to other therapies. This is why we have a multi-faceted program including an integrative scheme of drugs, diets, procedures, and medical care. By sensitizing the cancer, we are able to avoid using aggressive therapies that can destroy the patient's quality of life. It is time for physicians to consider how to use amygdalin in combination with conventional therapies at lower, non-aggressive dosages. Amygdalin, combined with vitamin C, can deplete glutathione and cysteine in tumor cells and make it possible to destroy the cancer with very low doses of chemotherapy, phytochemicals, UV light irradiation, and ozone. Though I have spoken out against the aggressive use of chemotherapy, it should be considered for use in low non-toxic doses when combined with amygdalin.

Scientific controversies sometimes take centuries or even millennia to resolve. When Copernicus published his "heliocentric" theory of the universe in 1543 it caused a hellish turmoil. He had to flee to Germany in order to escape being burned at the stake for suggesting such a blasphemous idea. But his 16th century non-fanatic and objective peers had well founded scientific concerns. They asked him, "If your doctrines are true, Venus would show phases like the moon." You see, at that time astrologers always saw Venus shining bright with the naked eye because the telescope had not been invented. He answered humbly, "You are right; I know not what to say; but God is good, and will in time find an answer to this objection." Almost a century passed when Galileo Galilei in 1633, looked through a telescope and saw the phases of Venus. Copernicus theory, that the earth circulates around the sun and not the other way around, was confirmed and he was vindicated.

Likewise, for decades scientists, in spite of the fact that there are many scientific publications about the antitumor effects of amygdalin, have had some founded and unfounded concerns, about the use of cyanide to treat cancer.

Amygdalin has a bright future using another technology being developed at the Imperial College in London. It can be used as a "prodrug." Scientists have found a way to attach amygdalin to a cancer-seeking antibody that will deliver it directly to the tumor and release the cyanide. Our plans at Oasis are to further develop the concept of amygdalin as a prodrug.

In the late 1980s and early 1990s, British scientists began study-ing the mechanism by which some plants use cyanide to defend them-selves from insects. They also studied its application in the treatment of cancer. Dr. Rowlinson-Busza, and Dr. Epenetos from the Imperial College in London, published an article in the journal *Applications in Clinical Oncology* titled "Cytotoxicity following specific activa-tion of amygdalin in monoclonal antibodies"[3] showing that cyanide is a potent antitumor agent.

The development of technology has led to the possibility of treating cancers by exploiting the differences between malignant and normal cells. The concept currently under investigation in England is the use of anti-bodies to carry enzymes to tumor cells, where they activate a prodrug. This is known as antibody-directed enzyme prodrug therapy (ADEPT). In this process, tumor-associated antibodies, directed against tumor an-tigens, are linked to enzymes and administered systemically. A prodrug is then administered and converted by the enzyme into an active cytotoxic agent at the tumor site. Therefore, the development of a prodrug system that activates an agent with a different mode of action and without any known resistance would be highly desirable.

A recent research project (Syrigos K et al, 1998)[4] studied a novel version of antibody-directed enzyme prodrug therapy, with the use of amygdalin as the prodrug. If amygdalin could be activated specifically at the tumor site, then malignant cells would be killed without the systemic toxicity usually associated with chemotherapy. The hydrolysis of amygdalin by the enzyme ß-glucosidase results in the release of the powerful poison cyanide.

The results of cytotoxicity studies demonstrate that amygdalin alone is virtually non-toxic having some cell killing effect only at high concentrations. The enzyme ß-glucosidase is also non-toxic, when amygdalin is not present. When amygdalin is exposed to the enzyme ß-glucosidase, either in its free form or conjugated to an antibody, then its toxicity is considerably increased 25-40 fold.

Additionally in this study, amygdalin was found to be signifi-cantly more toxic in vitro in combination with specific antibody enzyme conjugate than with the unconjugated enzyme at the same concentration. This finding is explained by the fact that, as antibody ß-glucosidase conjugate is bound to the cancer cells, the activity of amygdalin increased up to 115 fold in a dose-dependent fashion. Most of the cyanide is released in the vicinity of the tumor cell diffusing through the cell membrane, causing cancer cell death.

Using this technique in 1999, Professor Monica Hughes, chair of the Plant Molecular Genetics at the University of Newcastle upon Tyne in the North East of England, has treated brain tumors in rats obtaining 100 percent tumor destruction without any side effects.

The September 7, 2000 headline of the UK's newspaper *Independent* read, "Magic Bullet of Cyanide Could Kill Cancer Cells". The article goes on to state, "Cancer patients of the future could be treated with a powerful 'magic bullet' that attacks tumours with a cyanide cocktail derived from the cassava plant, scientists disclosed yesterday at the British Association's annual meeting…"

In 2002, Kousparou, Epenetos, and Deonarain,[5] from the Imperial College in London reported in the *International Journal of Cancer* that, "Antibody Guided Enzyme Therapy of cancer cells producing cyanide results in necrosis of targeted cells" without damage to the normal cells.

When I met with Dr. Mahendra Deonarain and Dr. Epenetos in the Department of Biochemistry at the Imperial College, Dr. Deonarain said "what we have done is to generate cyanide in the cancer cells only," and Dr. Epenetos asserted, "cyanide is the best anticancer agent nature has to offer."

These studies in England vindicated my father's many decades of ostracism and humiliation. My dad rejoiced when he read the reports. I credit him with this pioneering work but I'm sure, if he were alive today he would tell me that if a "magic bullet" were ever to be found, it would be one made by God, found in nature. Could it be cyanide-rich apricot seeds? As impressive as the laetrile record is, amygdalin is only the first of a multi-pronged attack against the disease. A magic bullet will never address all of the variables related to cancer.

It is not enough merely to launch a direct attack against the "muscle" of cancer. It is equally important to attack the "brains" of cancer. If the tumor cell is the muscle, then the programming that dictates tumor cell behavior is the brains of the disease. This is why the use of pancreatic enzymes is so important.

There is a key difference between normal cells and tumor cells. Normal cells are programmed to grow rapidly in their juvenile state, but the program changes as they mature, eventually dictating some function for the cells to serve within the body. Tumor cells never mature. Their programming freezes in the juvenile state, and they continue to reproduce at an alarming rate and send trophoblasts through the body's circulatory system in order to spread to other areas. So, how do pancreatic enzymes address this problem?

Enzymes are essential biochemical units that play a necessary role in virtually all of the functions of every organ system in the body. Life as we know it could not exist without the action of enzymes.

Enzymes are catalysts, substances that accelerate and precipitate the biochemical reactions that control life's processes in the organism. Each enzyme has a specific function in the body that no other enzyme can fulfill.

Digestive enzymes are secreted along the gastrointestinal tract and break down foods, enabling the nutrients to be absorbed into the blood stream for use in various bodily functions.

Proteases (proteolytic enzymes), one of the three main categories of digestive enzymes, are found in the stomach juices, pancreatic juices, and intestinal juices. Proteolytic enzymes help to digest proteins.

Plant extracts with a high content of proteolytic enzymes have been used for years in traditional medicine. Besides proteolytic enzymes from plants, such as papain and bromelain obtained from papayas and pineapples respectively, "modern" enzyme therapy additionally includes proteolytic pancreatic enzymes, such as chymotrypsin, tripsin, pepsin and pancreatin.[6] Proteolytic enzymes are used primarily to aid digestion and absorption of proteins contained in food. In addition to aiding digestion, proteolytic enzymes have analgesic, anti-inflammatory, antithrombotic, fibrinolytic, immune modulating, and edema-reducing properties.[7]

Results from recent research studies showed that proteolytic enzymes can produce great benefits in cancer therapy by improving the quality of life, reducing both the signs and symptoms of the disease and the adverse effects caused by radiotherapy and chemotherapy,[8] and prolonging the survival time.[9]

Proteolytic enzymes act as immunomodulators by raising the impaired immunocytotoxicity of leukocytes against tumor cells from patients and by inducing the production of distinct cytokines such as tumor necrosis factor, interleukin (IL)-1, IL-6 and IL-8.[10]

There are reports on animal experiments claiming an anti-metastatic efficacy of proteolytic enzymes associated with inhibition of growth and invasiveness of tumor cells.[11]

All these antitumoral activities do not depend on the proteolytic activity of enzymes, but of their effects on the modulation of immune functions, including the anti-inflammatory activities and their potential to accelerate wound healing.[12]

Proteolytic enzymes are also used in the treatment of pancreatic insufficiency, cystic fibrosis, digestive problems, viral infections, surgical traumas, autoimmune disorders and sports injuries.[13]

Enzyme therapy can significantly clear "immune complexes" (combinations of antibodies and antigens) from the body. When the body is incapable of releasing these immune complexes, an inflammatory process begins that can lead to serious disease, often of the autoimmune type.[14] Dramatic results have been reported with the use of enzyme therapy in such diseases as rheumatoid arthritis, multiple-sclerosis, and systemic lupus erythematosus.[15]

Another important part of our treatment strategy is to cut off tumor supply lines. Think of the armies of ancient Greece laying siege to enemy cities in an effort to starve them into surrender. The siege of a tumor is accomplished with the use of shark cartilage.

Shark cartilage inhibits the growth of blood vessels which feed growing tumors, thereby restricting the vitality of the tumor. In other words, shark cartilage puts cancer on a starvation diet. In a clinical trial conducted by Dr. Ernesto Contreras and Dr. William Lane, it was noted that tumors frequently experienced significant reduction in size within one to three months of the initial treatment. [16]

Shark cartilage contains mucopolysaccharides, glycoproteins, collagen and glycosaminoglycans, including chondroitin sulfate A, B, and C. Due to these components, shark cartilage:

- Accelerates wound healing. Glycosaminoglycans are responsible of this effect.[17]
- Has a powerful anti-inflammatory activity due to its mucopolysaccharide components.
- Stimulates the immune system.[18]
- Contains anti-angiogenesis factors (glycoproteins) that inhibit the formation of new blood vessels.[19]

The growth and metastasis of malignant tumors are dependent on angiogenesis, the formation of new blood vessels, to meet the progressively increasing demand for oxygen and essential nutrients. Angiogenesis and anti-angiogenesis are multifactorial and counter-acting mechanisms that involve a number of stimulatory and inhibitory factors secreted by tumor cells, non-neoplastic cells within the tumor, and by macrophages, mast cells, and endothelial cells. Dr. Folkman first proposed inhibition of angiogenesis as a mechanism for controlling tumor growth in 1971.[20]

Recently there is a dramatic increase in the development and use of anti-angiogenic agents for the treatment of cancer. The first reported biological inhibition of angiogenesis was bovine cartilage. The most potent variety of cartilage appears to be that derived from shark. Two glycoproteins, sphyrnastatin 1 and 2, have been isolated from shark cartilage and reported to have strong anti-angiogenic activity and to inhibit tumor neovascularisation.[21]

There has been considerable debate concerning the use of shark cartilage as an anti-angiogenic agent in cancer therapy. Evidence has been presented indicating that shark cartilage can inhibit blood vessel formation. Tumor neovascualrization is considerably reduced in rabbit corneas by implanted copolymer pellets containing shark cartilage extract. Considerable skepticism has been voiced with regard to oral administration of shark cartilage owing to digestive breakdown of cartilage within the gastrointestinal tract. However, results from recent studies demonstrated that oral shark cartilage has significant anti-angiogenic activity, suggesting that this skepticism is unfounded.[22] Researchers demonstrated that shark cartilage is effective in inhibiting tumor growth and increasing survival rates in animals and patients with cancer. In one of the studies with tumor-bearing rats, shark cartilage administered orally extended the survival time by 30 percent.[23]

Researchers from a recent study concluded that oral shark cartilage does not abolish carcinogenesis but delays progression in renal tumors in mice.[24] Dupont E et al., 1997[25] showed that a liquid extract from shark cartilage inhibited blood vessel formation and endothelial cell proliferation in vitro. The liquid extract from shark cartilage showed in vitro antitumor activity against human breast cancer, human ovarian adenocarcinoma, and human epidermoid carcinoma. This agent inhibited tumor-cell growth in murine mammary carcinoma and reduced metastases in the Lewis lung carcinoma model in mice.[26]

In a clinical trial in the USA, 50 percent of patients who took dried cartilage powder daily, reported improvements in quality of life and appetite, and reduction in pain.[27]

Let's summarize before we go on. With amygdalin, we deliver cyanide to attack the malignant cells and the amygdalin sensitizes the tumor to other anticancer treatments. The pancreatic enzymes are used to increase the activity of the immune system's anticancer cells. We use shark cartilage to cut off the tumors supply of new blood vessesls. The next step is to derail cancer's transportation system. We use emulsified vitamin A because it travels the same paths as cancer cells do and it has antitumor qualities.

Studies, initiated in Germany, tried to determine why Norwegian sailors had very low incidences of lung cancer though most had smoked cigarrettes since early childhood. The answer was found in their diet. They consumed large quantities of raw fish liver which is rich in vitamin A. The logical deduction was that high doses of the vitamin A prevented the growth of lung cancer in long-term smokers.

Researchers developed a high concentration A-Emulsion in which one drop contains 15,000 International Units (IU) of vitamin A. Researchers were able to administer, in gradually progressive doses, over a million IU per day without producing toxic effects. Emulsified vitamin A has a number of beneficial effects. In doses of 100,000 to 300,000 IU per day, it works as a potent immune-stimulant. In doses of 500,000 to 1,000,000 IU per day, it serves as a potent antitumor agent, traveling through the lymphatic system to tumor sites throughout the body.

The combined effect of amygdalin, pancreatic enzymes, shark cartilage and vitamin A emulsion is impressive. When you attack disease from every available angle, you afford the patient the maximum chance of recovery. This is why these four agents comprise the foundation of my father's "Metabolic Therapy."

There are even more exciting things on the horizon. Let's look at some new therapies we have been researching, developing, and using since the 1990s. These include ozone therapy, ultraviolet light and other agents found in nature.

# CHAPTER TEN

## *Something In The Air*

A nephew of mine told a story recently about an adventure he had when he was in college at San Diego State University. He and a friend were hanging out on a Friday night. They had driven to Pacific Beach to grab a late night bite to eat and then stopped by a local pool hall to shoot a few racks of nine-ball before closing time. When they piled into my nephew's VW beetle and headed home, it was almost two 'o' clock in the morning.

Halfway home, they changed freeways and began to drive past a rough area of the city. It was right at that moment that the car decided to run out of gas without warning. I say without warning because my nephew asserts that the gas gauge, speedometer, and odometer did not work in this vehicle. Remember, this is a college student's car. Well, there they stood on the shoulder of the road at two in the morning, the sound of police cars and circling helicopters just a little too close.

Five minutes passed and neither of these geniuses could think of a way out of the mess. This was before the days of cell phones, mind you. Suddenly, a gigantic four-wheel-drive passed by, swerving onto the shoulder about a hundred yards ahead. Its taillights flared and it backed up to them. I was not comforted by the fact that the gun-rack in the window was empty. The driver's door opened and the meanest-looking man my nephew had ever seen stepped out of the truck.

His full beard covered half of his massive chest. He wore a battered and torn biker vest and a pair of greasy blue jeans. The thick boots on his feet punished the ground as he strode around the car to where the boys stood. My initial assessment was that this was a self-proclaimed freedom fighter, what you might call a "free radical." My nephew tried to remember if he had ever filled out a last will and testament. "Got a problem?" the man growled.

"No. No problem," the boys spluttered.

"Aren't you broke down?" he said, glancing at the car.

"Oh that," my nephew answered, "Yeah. We're out of gas."

"Be right back," he rumbled and he was gone. His four-by roared up the freeway, over the crest of the hill, and was gone. Five minutes later, he was back with a three-gallon can of gasoline. He emptied the can into their car, shook their hands, and drove off again. The boys were absolutely stunned. Help had come from the unlikeliest of places.

While it is true that the metabolic therapy we have pioneered has helped many people, there is a limitation to it. You see, metabolic therapy is a program designed to achieve long-term results. It takes time to establish long-lasting results. This means that we rarely witness tumor regression during the patient's initial treatment.

When a patient is facing cancer, they want to see immediate results. This is why many patients turn to chemotherapy. While chemotherapy may shrink tumors very quickly, the long-term results have been less than impressive. In fact, they have been pretty frightening.

Yet, we understand that the emotional health of a patient can be improved when there is evidence of immediate progress. We knew we could not turn to conventional therapies for those results because of the damage they cause to a patient's immune system. We began exploring other options. Just like my nephew, we discovered that help sometimes comes from the unlikeliest of places.

When most people hear the word ozone, they think of a protective layer of our atmosphere but aren't really sure what it is beyond that. Ozone is oxygen but with the molecular structure $O_3$ instead of $O_2$. This additional molecule makes ozone a highly reactive oxidant. If inhaled, ozone can do some serious damage to our bodies. However, there is an application of this substance that is very therapeutic. But first, let's take a closer look at ozone.

In nature, ozone has a good side and a bad side. In the stratosphere, it acts as a shield, deflecting harmful UV irradiation. However, in the troposphere, ozone is a major component of the smog that harms humans, animals, and plants. When we breathe it, ozone can cause serious pulmonary and systemic side effects because it is such a powerful oxidant.[1]

It has been shown that ozone possesses broad-spectrum antimicrobial activity.[2] This means that it fights the bacteria that cause infection. In the First World War, it was used by medics to save the lives of wounded soldiers suffering from gaseous gangrene. Today ozonated solutions and ozonated oils are still used to treat wounds and a host of infections. Ozone therapies are used to treat fistulae, abscesses, ulcers, gingivitis, stomatitis, and osteomyelitis. In addition, ozone has been widely used in sewage treatment and water purification processes because it is such an effective bacterial scavenger.[3]

On the world scene, ozone therapy became an alternative medical approach in 1954, when Wehrly and Steinbart first described its application. They found that while the human respiratory tract reacts very negatively to ozone, human blood does not. In fact, when exposed to appropriate ozone concentrations, our blood tames the strong oxidant properties of ozone, thus eliminating any acute side effects. The benefits derived from this therapy are staggering.

Oasis doctors know that ozonation of the blood improves the exchange of oxygen in the blood, activates the immune system, and increases the efficiency of the antioxidant system. What is most exciting to us is how these three things combine to effectively retard or reverse tumor growth. It is obvious to our doctors that ozone is useful in the treatment of degenerative diseases like cancer.

Over the last seven years, doctors at Oasis have advanced the use of ozone therapy, the results have been extraordinary. Our patients have experienced measurable tumor reduction quickly, sometimes in as little as two weeks. For long-term results, we still believe that metabolic therapy is vital, but it is wonderful to get fast results, too. Let me explain how ozone therapy is administered.

Autohemotherapy is the process of bringing small quantities of blood into contact with ozone.[4] This ozone therapy is performed each year on several hundred thousand patients around the world, mostly in Russia, Poland, Greece, Germany, Switzerland, Italy, Austria, Belgium and Cuba.[5] The medical ozone used in this therapy is an $O_2/O_3$ mixture with a low ozone concentration. The ozone generators used to produce this mixture are incredibly precise.[6]

Autohemotherapy is typically performed in one of two ways. The standard technique is to withdraw 150-250 ml of blood and expose it to a $O_2/O_3$ mixture at a specified ozone concentration, followed by intravenous reinfusion of this blood into the patient.[7] At the Oasis of Hope, we have the option of running an extracorporeal loop to ozonate all of the patient's blood. This second technique involves automatically running the blood through a continuous recirculating device which mixes ozone and blood in a closed loop before reinfusing it.[8]

The results from two very recent studies proved the safety and effectiveness of the ozonation of blood in humans. No significant changes in blood chemistry or other parameters were found. The patients felt no particular sensations during treatment. The treatment session was followed by a feeling of well-being and euphoria, lasting several hours. Most importantly, there was a total lack of side effects. The authors conclude that blood ozonation is clinically valid, without side effects and that there are at least four areas, namely infectious diseases, vascular disorders, degenerative diseases (particularly metastatic cancer), and pathologies related to immune depression, where this treatment could be useful when orthodox therapies have failed.[9] All of these factors fall within the principles embraced by Oasis doctors.

So, how does the ozone actually work? Personally, I am fascinated by the cascade of effects ozone provokes when it is introduced into the bloodstream. Ozone decomposes in blood and interacts immediately with several substances, namely fatty acids, cholesterols, proteins, and carbohydrates.[10]   When the ozone decomposes a series of reactive oxygen species are quickly produced, the most important of which is hydrogen peroxide ($H_2O_2$).

A sudden rise in $H_2O_2$ concentration triggers very different biochemical activity depending upon the type of cell the $H_2O_2$ penetrates.[11]   If the $H_2O_2$ penetrates red cells and endothelial cells, three things happen. First, there is an increase in the delivery and release of oxygen by red cells toward the tissues.[12]   Then, in areas of the system that were constricted, endothelial cells enhance release of nitric oxide (NO)[13] resulting in dilation of blood vessels and improving oxygen flow.[14]   Finally, the formation of new blood vessels (angiogenesis) is inhibited due to the improvement of oxygenation in the neoplastic tissue. Remember, tumors feed on blood vessels. Thus, anything that reduces the formation of blood vessels helps to restrain tumor growth.

When $H_2O_2$ penetrates cells known as leukocytes, it induces the production of specialized biological assassins called cytokines. These include interleukins, interferon, and tumor necrosis factor.[15] The cytokines launch an array of immune functions, such as macrophages and neutrophils, which slow tumor growth and metastasis.[16]

The presence of $H_2O_2$ in the blood increases the efficiency with which the body eliminates oxidants. We know that persistent oxidative stress from free radicals, or oxidants, is at the root of degenerative diseases like cancer. Countless findings show that aging, chronic viral infections, cancer, autoimmune diseases, and neurodegenerative diseases are all accompanied by a reduction in the body's ability to detoxify itself properly.

Without question, ozone therapy will rapidly become an essential tool for oncologists and an integral part of comprehensive treatment programs. Over the next few years, Oasis doctors will continue to refine the use of ozone therapy. I expect even more dramatic results.

# CHAPTER ELEVEN

## *Seeing The Light*

We live in the age of invention. The push to continually bring a new product into the marketplace is intense in the business world. Yet, it is not the steady stream of gadgets that really grabs my attention. It is the inventors who have always baffled me. I have always wondered what it must be like to see the world as they see it.

What was it that made the first rocket scientist think, as he gazed up at the moon, "I can get there." At what point in his life did Ben Franklin watch a lightning storm and think, "I can catch one of those." It is that mindset that fascinates me.

The 20th century was a time of amazing innovation in the medical industry. These technological advancements particularly interest me. For one, my practice and my patients benefit from them. The men behind such innovations have earned my respect and admiration because they are willing to take such radical departures from the mainstream in search of new hope. One such technological advancement is the use of ultraviolet light as an antitumor agent.

Researchers began to consider the use of ultraviolet light to treat disease in the 1870s. At the time, scientists understood that ultraviolet light was extremely efficient at eliminating bacteria. Dr. Neils Ryberg Finsen and several other prominent physicians suggested the use of ultraviolet light to destroy infectious organisms in the blood. Finsen was one of the first researchers to irradiate blood with ultraviolet light. In 1903, he won the Nobel Prize in Medicine for his work treating the blood of 300 lupus patients with ultraviolet light.[1]

The next major innovation in the therapy came in 1928, when American researchers E. Knott and V. Hancock used a device that made extracorporeal ultraviolet blood irradiation (UVBI) possible. They conducted the first successful treatment of septic infection with the therapy. Later work revealed that ultraviolet light has a positive influence on the immune, respiratory, and hormonal systems. So, why has it been regarded as a new therapy?

Sadly, the answer is all too clear. A host of new antibiotics and vaccines were introduced in the 1950s. The medical industry was so enthusiastic to use these products that the UVBI device was placed on a shelf. What is most disappointing about this is that for many illnesses, like hepatitis and pneumonia, UVBI treatment was clearly superior. Thankfully, interest in UVBI therapy was rekindled two decades later in Russia.[2] Let me explain how the actual treatment is administered.

There are two pieces of equipment needed to administer extra corporeal UVBI therapy. The first, obviously, is a source of ultraviolet light. The second is an irradiation chamber made from quartz glass, which is permeable for ultraviolet radiation.

The standard procedure is known as the Knott technique.[3] First, doctors draw 1.5 ml of blood per pound of body weight, never exceeding 250 ml. The blood is drawn into a transfusion flask containing a small amount of an anticoagulant such as heparin or citrate. This additive prevents clots from forming in the bottle or the tubing.

Next, the blood is pumped through the special tubing at a controlled rate. The currently acceptable rate is approximately 0.5 ml/sec. The blood flows through an irradiation chamber, called a cuvette, where it is exposed for up to ten seconds to a controlled amount of ultraviolet irradiation. The specialized lamps used generate a therapeutic band of ultraviolet light.

Finally, when the correct amount of blood has been irradiated and stored in a flask, the flow is reversed and the blood is irradiated a second time when reinfused into the body. However, at the Oasis of Hope, an extra step is added. Blood is ozonized just before reinfusion because the combined effectiveness of the two therapies is greater than if they were administered separately.

The entire procedure takes thirty minutes. This includes ten minutes for set-up and ten minutes for clean up. The new devices at Oasis contain disposable crystal reaction chambers and disposable tubing to avoid the use of potentially contaminated materials.

The treatment variables can be tailored to the needs of each patient. Some patients receive treatment daily, others weekly. Some patients receive a course of three sessions, others as many as eight. Some patients treat 100 ml of blood each session, others up to 250 ml. Yet, the best thing about the therapy is how it works.

During the early years of UVBI therapy, Knott and his associates sought to explain how the treatment obtains its therapeutic effects. Research has identified two probable modes. The first explanation is that the ultraviolet irradiation destroys bacteria and viruses in the extracted blood and creates a kind of "vaccination effect." In other words, when the irradiated blood returns to the body, the immune system identifies the dead bacteria and viruses in it. It then seeks out and destroys the same bacteria and viruses in the non-irradiated blood in the rest of the body.[4]

The second explanation is that when the small fraction of irradiated blood is re-infused, it begins to spread throughout the entire volume of blood in the body. These irradiated blood cells give off secondary radiation. The secondary radiation destroys viruses, bacteria, and toxins. In addition, it activates white blood cells.[5]

Strong evidence suggests that UVBI therapy has a prophylactic action against cancer. A study in East Germany measured the number of mutations produced by chromosomes. After six sessions of UVBI therapy, researchers found that the number of chromosomal mutations diminished. These doctors believe that UVBI therapy can actually stimulate DNA repair.[6]

Compared to orthodox treatments, UVBI therapy is extremely safe. A Russian study of 2,380 sessions of UVBI therapy revealed that only 1.3 percent of patients experienced side effects and that they were mild.[7] The benefits clearly out-weigh the slight potential of mild side effects.

The next major advancement in the therapy came in 1987 when a new form of UVBI termed extracorporeal photopheresis (ECP) therapy was introduced. This procedure entails combining a special type of ultraviolet light with a photoactivatable substance called 8-MOP. ECP therapy was originally used to treat patients with cutaneous T-Cell lymphoma (TCL).[8] Today, ECP remains the only FDA approved tumor-targeting selective immunotherapy for the treatment of TCL, and it is in use in over 150 centers worldwide.[9] The treatment is also used to treat a wide variety of diseases like systemic sclerosis, rheumatoid arthritis, and lupus.[10]

One of the key components to this therapy is the 8-MOP, a naturally occurring substance produced in large quantity by the common weed Queen Anne's lace.[11] Smaller quantities can be found in a variety of fruits and vegetables, such as figs, limes, parsnips, and celery. Scientists recognize that 8-MOP is activated by ultraviolet energy. When activated, 8-MOP cross-links with cellular DNA.[12]

When the 8-MOP is activated by UV Light and does not react against a target chemical, it returns to be a harmless substance, and is eliminated from the body within a day. 8-MOP is only effective after direct activation by ultraviolet energy and that exposure takes place outside the body. In other words, 8-MOP targets only those cells simultaneously exposed to both the drug and the activating light. Therefore, because the body's organs have not been exposed to the ultraviolet light, they are spared any adverse reactions from the 8-MOP activation.

Other toxic effects commonly associated with DNA binding agents, such as bone marrow suppression, hair loss, or mucosal erosions are also not encountered. In addition, opportunistic infections are avoided because the therapy is so precise. This is not true of conventional systemic chemotherapy, which typically induces generalized suppression of the immune system. These features make ECP the most "controllable" potent therapy currently in clinical use.

The therapy itself involves several steps. First, white blood cells are harvested extracorporeally and bathed in plasma containing 8-MOP, which has been circulated through an ultraviolet irradiation field.[13] Then, the solution is re-infused into the body. The mechanical stress to which the monocytes were subjected to during the procedure induces white blood cells known as monocytes to convert into dendritic antigen presenting cells. These are the cells which initiate immune reactions by identifying targets for the immune system.[14] In regard to cancer, dendritic cells initiate an antitumor response from the immune system by identifying malignant cells as a target.[15]

Treatment with ECP therapy also increases the production of the cytokines the immune system uses to kill malignant cells. Specifically, the therapy increases production of interferon and interleukin-2.[16] Without question, the most important anticancer cytokine is interleukin-2. A cancer immunotherapy requires the transfer of tumor-distinctive antigens from malignant cells to "professional" antigen-presenting cells, like dendritic cells, to initiate clinically relevant antitumor responses from the immune system, like the production of interleukin.[17]

At Oasis Hospital we combine ozonization with UV irradiation of the blood. On one hand, irridiation of the blood begins the process of transforming monocytes into immature dendritic cells. On the other, it is known that oxidative stress generated during ozonization and UV irradiation of the blood at the moment of reinfusion promotes maturation of dendritic cells.[18]

There is a recent modification to standard ECP therapy called transimmunization therapy (TI). This is a way of tailor-making the therapy to individual patients. The first major difference is that the white blood cells are cultured overnight after exposure to the 8-MOP and ultraviolet light.[19] The white blood cells called monocytes transform immature dendritic cells.[20] These immature dendritic cells are aggressive and can internalize apoptotic cancer cells. So, the white blood cells are cultured overnight with a solution of dead cancer cells, removed from the patient in surgery. The immature dendritic cells ingest these cancer cells stimulating a "specific" antitumor immunity. When the antigen-loaded dendritic cells mature, they are intravenously returned to the patient and stimulate a "personalized antitumor vaccine."[21]

The various applications of ultraviolet light as an antitumor agent are exciting. My hope is that more and more cancer treatment facilities will incorporate emerging therapies like UVBI, ECP, and TI into their programs. These therapies are incredibly effective and do not destroy the immune system or compromise the emotional health of the patient.

# CHAPTER TWELVE

## *It's Emotional*

Let me relate a story to you and see if you don't identify with it. A few weeks ago, I got up early to drive my son to school in the morning. We sat down in the kitchen together and ate a quiet breakfast and looked over his Yugi-O trading card collection. We put on our jackets and went out to the car. There was a light fog that morning and the air was crisp and cool. I felt happy and relaxed as I buckled him into the passenger seat.

We pulled out of the driveway and made our way to the edge of our neighborhood. I soon found myself stopped at a traffic signal. The light turned green and I began to make a left-hand turn. By instinct, I glanced to my right and saw him coming. I barely had time to cut my turn short before a Jeep Cherokee barreled through the red light and blew by the passenger side at fifty plus.

I leaned on the horn for a split second and then completed the turn. As I proceeded down the street, I noticed that the Jeep was slowing down. At the next intersection it came to a complete stop even though the light was green. "He's waiting for me," I thought. Sure enough, when I pulled up a little behind him, I could see him through his rear window gesturing angrily at me with a particular finger.

I couldn't believe it! This guy runs a red light, almost kills my son, and he's mad at *me* because I honked at him once? I drove around him and within a few blocks he lost interest and went about his merry way. I, on the other hand, was a wreck. My adrenaline raced for easily thirty minutes and I was in a sour mood for the rest of the day. I had difficulty concentrating in the office that morning, I stared distastefully at my lunch, and I was still keyed up about it that evening as I related the story to my wife and discovered that I had a splitting headache.

What happened to me was totally and completely natural. Common sense and science both tell us that our emotions have an impact on our physiology. There are a number of physiological responses that correspond to each specific emotion. You feel afraid and your heart races. You experience anxiety and you begin to sweat. Each emotion triggers the release of specific hormones and the body reacts in a predictable fashion to the increased production of these substances. Often these emotions manifest into a physical ailment, like a racking headache.

The last component of a truly comprehensive treatment program is the alteration of the patient's lifestyle. This aspect of treatment is one of the gaping deficiencies in oncological practice today. The current trend of separating body, mind, and spirit in modern medicine is something that must be changed if patients are to truly achieve wellness.

So, where do we begin? First, doctor and patient must acknowledge the importance of working toward a positive state of emotional health. Both sides must agree that any emotion that has a negative impact on the immune system must be worked through fully and eliminated as much as possible. I firmly believe that, in some cases, cancer may set roots in an existing emotional imbalance.

This is where a thorough counseling program can provide tremendous benefit. Daniel Kennedy has been working to further develop the counseling program at Oasis. We understand that patients often need help working through many of the emotional stages that a cancer crises induces.

The first stage is shock. Unless it has happened to them, the average person has no idea what it is like to sit in a doctor's office and have him or her look them in the eye and say, "You have cancer." I have had to help people out of their chair because the shock completely freezes them. Breaking that news is never a pleasant experience. It is like strapping a hundred pound weight onto a person's back. The news generates shock because it is usually unexpected. Surprisingly, few people will share the news with loved ones until the shock wears off. It is critical to help patients through this stage because every cancer patient needs a solid support structure of family and friends to rally around them.

The second stage, called denial, can often accompany the first. The experience of facing the possibility of one's own mortality is so devastating that many people are unable to acknowledge the reality of the situation. These people will either openly or secretly accuse their physician of incompetence. They may adopt a cavalier attitude, thinking, "This isn't that big of a deal," or, "I can beat this thing easy." Needless to say, it is incredibly dangerous to underestimate the seriousness of the threat cancer poses. The first step to getting a patient into a comprehensive treatment program is helping them to acknowledge the importance of doing so.

The third stage, fear, can also accompany the first. Sometimes seconds after hearing the diagnosis, a person can be overwhelmed with fear. In the case of cancer, this fear is often twofold. The patient not only experiences the fear of death but also the fear of the suffering associated with the disease and conventional treatment programs. In my own experience, I have witnessed strong evidence that fear is the stronghold of cancer. I believe that this emotion can literally fuel the progression of the tumor. Helping a patient to fully embrace the hope of healing is a critical step in the effort to establish positive emotional health.

The fourth stage, grief, occurs when the reality of the situation has time to settle. There comes a point, sometimes in the middle of very successful treatment, when the patient is overwhelmed with sadness. The possibility of missing out on life and the lives of loved ones is a crushing reality. While this emotion is completely normal and understandable, it can be dangerous if unaddressed. The grief can be so intense, it can cause a person to isolate themself from the very support structure they desperately need. Often, a person will close themselves off to others in an effort to spare the people they love pain and suffering. However, the emotional burden of a fight with cancer must be shared, because it is too intense for any one person to bear.

The fifth stage, anger, often comes after the patient is fully engaged in the battle with the disease. Patients find themselves asking, "Why me, God?" Many patients are tempted to suppress these questions as inappropriate. I couldn't disagree more. In fact, I firmly believe that obtaining the answer to that question is extremely important. Swallowing the desire for that answer will only breed resentment and cripple a patient's faith.

The sixth stage is connected to the fifth. If a person attempts to work through the "why me" question without support, they may experience feelings of guilt or inadequacy. They may think, "I deserve this somehow," "This is my fault," or "I'm not getting better because I lack faith." Again, these feelings are normal and understandable, but dangerous if not worked through fully. Patients need help coming to terms with the fragile nature of life and the fine line between health and illness.

The seventh stage of acceptance and resolve is the goal. When a patient reaches this stage, I am confident that they are in a positive emotional state that does not compromise the opportunity for healing. These patients accept their situation and have decided to be proactive about seeking a solution.

Remember, the first step to altering lifestyle is to secure a healthy emotional state. One of our goals at Oasis is to guide patients through the negative emotions of the first six stages to a place of peace and confidence in the seventh stage. Let's look at a variety of therapies that can compliment a strong counseling program and support a patient emotionally.

# CHAPTER THIRTEEN

## *Mind Medicine*

Our history to some measure defines us, in much the same way as the roads we have traveled are connected to our current location. This is certainly true of my father. His character as a physician was shaped by his childhood experiences. His character, in turn, shaped mine.

When the Mexican revolution began, my father's family lost everything.[1] They were a "riches to rags" story. As a young boy, he learned hardship first hand. The loss of comfort and security was devastating to all members of his family, but it absolutely broke his father. My grandfather abandoned my grandmother and left her to fend for herself and five children. He died shortly thereafter.

My grandmother became a state teacher. Today, teachers in California threaten to strike year after year because of low wages, but imagine a teacher in Mexico City in the 1930s! She barely made enough to survive. Yet, there was a life and vitality to that family that defies explanation.

Somehow, in the midst of those years of hardship, my father discovered the healing power of music and humor. He learned from experience that these things were medicine to the soul and kept him motivated. He learned that life was better when he heard the music in the world around him and saw the humor in the situations he encountered in everyday life. He worked hard to internalize these lessons.

When my father, with the help of an uncle, was admitted into the military medical school, he arrived ready to study with books under one arm, his guitar under the other, and a smile as his umbrella. He had learned that music and humor could bring smiles to the faces of those who lived under difficult circumstances. He knew he would see difficult circumstances as a medical student.

My father graduated from medical school in 1939 and practiced medicine for almost twenty-five years before opening the Oasis of Hope. He arrived to work everyday with patient files under one arm, a guitar under the other, and a smile as his umbrella. Nothing had changed. In the mornings, he consulted with patients. In the afternoons he would gather them together to talk about hope, love, and faith. He would play songs for his patients. He would take requests. He invited them to sing along. He offered to put their original lyrics to music.

My father studied joke books so that he could help his patients laugh. He had excellent comic timing and the jokes were pretty funny, but that wasn't what made people laugh the most. What really made them laugh was the fact that the comedian wore a lab coat and a stethoscope. I never realized the impression that made on people until recently.

A former patient of his from years ago pulled me aside recently. "You know what I remember about your father?" she asked, tugging at my sleeve. "He made me laugh…really laugh." She smiled, "What do you get when you mix onions and beans?" I shrugged my shoulders. "Tear gas! Your dad told me that joke," she said. We shared the laugh together.

My father had a kind word, a song, a joke, and a hug for his patients. When patients were scheduled to leave the hospital, my father would go to their room to sing one last song with them before they left for home. I have never seen a doctor love his patients like my father.

It was the true love for his profession and his patients that made Dr. Ernesto Contreras, Sr. much more than a physician. He was a healer. His legacy lives through the Oasis of Hope staff today. We continue to love our patients in word, song, and laughter. We understand that the alteration of the patient's lifestyle is rooted in their emotional well-being. Following in our founder's footsteps, we provide activities, beyond our counseling program, that promote excellent emotional health.

There is no question that music speaks to our hearts in a way mere words can not. Paul Simon once talked about the song *Only Living Boy In New York* and commented that he liked the particular chord progression he chose to transition to the chorus of the song because studies reveal that it evokes tears. When I read that, I was fascinated. I had owned the record *Bridge Over Troubled Water* as a kid and that song always moved me to tears right at that spot. The fact that music can elicit particular emotions makes music a powerful tool in the hands of a physician.

Clinical research indicates that music can positively influence the respiratory system, the circulatory system, the immune system, and the endocrine system. Music can slow your respiratory rate. Music can lower your blood pressure. Music can bolster your body's defense mechanisms. Music can stimulate the production of endorphins.[2] Couple these effects with the emotional benefits and you'll agree that more doctors should prescribe music for their patients.

Most people are aware that each type of music affects their emotions differently. For example, when the teenage boy next door is playing music that sounds like a cat being dragged behind a noisy cement truck, I tend to pull my hair out by the roots. Conversely, when I listen to music I enjoy, I often relax and breathe easier. Teaching patients to incorporate music into their lives helps them shift focus off of the pain and stress that accompany a battle with cancer.

The first time I listened to Bill Cosby talk about his adventures with his brother Russell, I cried. Tears rolled down my face because my stomach hurt from laughing so hard. At one point, I had to stop the recording because I couldn't breathe. I actually thought, "If I don't hit the stop button and calm down, I am going to die." I pictured my parents walking into my room and finding my body on the floor, hands on my stomach, a smile plastered to my face. I had never been exposed to comic genius like that before. Bill Cosby introduced me to the notion that there are people who are truly gifted at making people laugh.

Do you know there is healing power in laughter? Dr. Norman Cousins[3] knew. When he was diagnosed with a degenerative disease, he checked himself out of the hospital. He went home and cured himself by adopting a diet of healthy foods, juices, and humor. He didn't get weak medicine either. He didn't settle for the cheap laughs that so many films today embrace. He surrounded himself with comic genius; Chaplin, Laurel and Hardy, Lucy and Desi, Cosby, etc. He ate, drank, and was merry. His illness went away.

Don't chalk his success story up to luck, either. He knew what he was doing. He knew about the benefits of good diet and laughter. Laughter helps the body release endorphins, obtain oxygen, and relax tense muscles. Science proves it to be a healing force. At Oasis, we encourage patients to incorporate humor into their lifestyle. We watch videos featuring gifted comedians. We enlist the service of laughter therapist Shary Oden. We help patients discover the wide variety of opportunities for laughter in their day-to-day world. We believe the healing power of laughter can help restore a person to a healthy emotional state and help them maintain that balance.

Want to see something funny? Take a man in his forties and show him a box of your kid's Legos. Then, say that you need to make a phone call and leave the room for sixty seconds. When you return, he will be playing with the Legos. If he isn't, I will personally pay you a dollar. There is something about the act of creating something that draws humans as the moon draws water. This is why art therapy is so important. It satisfies the basic human need to be creative.[4]

Oasis is a house of art. Situated around the hospital are original sculptures and paintings. All of the pieces are related to healing and uplifting passages from scripture. In a number of places, including the *www.oasisofhope.com* Internet site, you can see some artwork done by patients during their stay at Oasis. Making an original work of art can bring happiness and peace. Creating and talking about art helps patients to cope better with the stress of battling disease.

I have a confession to make. My father and I did not invent music therapy, laughter therapy, or art therapy. Yet, these things make the Oasis of Hope a unique treatment center. Few cancer centers incorporate these therapies into the treatment approach even though countless clinical trials indicate the benefit they offer patients.

The objective of these therapies is not to create warm fuzzy feelings, but to restore the mind to a balanced emotional state. Science has confirmed the therapeutic value of these therapies and we have witnessed positive changes in the majority of our patients for over forty years. That history alone defines who we are at Oasis and who we will continue to be.

We have a vision of how to improve treatment outcomes for our patients over the next five years. Yes, we will continue our efforts on the medical front, but the revolution we are starting in our program is on the emotional and spiritual fronts. My father did so many things right being lead by intuition or promptings of the Spirit. When he started in 1963, there were not many studies if any that supported the medicinal value of emotional support, but today the science behind it is confirmed by hundreds of clinical trials. Now, there is enough data available to develop a treatment program that fully integrates therapies for the body, mind and spirit as my father envisioned over four decades ago.

Our starting point, or justification for investing in the design of a counseling program, is that if we can help patients manage negative emotions and transform them into positive emotions, a boost to their immune systems will result and their probability of overcoming the illness will increase. If negative thought processes are not adressed, they will continue to depress the immune system making it more difficult for the body to recover. Aside from the physical benefit, we are aiming to aid patients obtain peace and overcome the fear of cancer. Illness can rob people of the joy of life. Even if a person has cancer, or especially if a person has cancer, they can make the most of each day and enjoy it. But most people find it hard to celebrate life when they are paralyzed by the fear of imminent death or devastating treatment experiences. Emotional victory over cancer is priceless. Some patients have told me that they never lived life the way they wanted to until it was threatened by cancer. Once death loomed, they began to value each day and live to the fullest. But these are the patients that were not paralyzed by fear. I will share the stories of three such patients in the chapter entitled *Great Expectations*. In the previous chapter, I outlined the negative emotions most cancer patients experience including shock, denial, fear, guilt, inadequacy, anger, and resentment. Clinical studies demonstrate the correlation of negative emotions and improper immune function. Either the immune system can be depressed or it can be overactive which can be equally as destructive. A study by Ishihara, Makita, Imai, Hashimoto, and Nohara on patients with coronary heart disease concluded, "Psychological factors are considered to influence the immune response."[5] Another study published by researchers at the University of Wisconsin-Madison concluded that, "If you're sad or blue, you're more likely to get sick."[6] There is an abundance of clinical studies that confirm the link between negative emotions and improper immune function. At the same time, there are many studies confirming that positive emotions enhance immune function. Bennett, Zeller, Rosenberg, and McCann wrote, "Laughter may reduce stress and improve NK cell activity. As low NK cell activity is linked to decreased disease resistance and increased morbidity in people with cancer and HIV disease, laughter may be a useful cognitive-behavioral intervention."[7] Another study indicates that, "Positive mood states and mirthful laughter enhance various aspects of immune functions." [8]

We have formed a group of advisors including psychologists, ministers and counselors/psychotherapists to help oversee the formation of our program. Together we have defined the main theories, principles and techniques that will be utilized in a group setting to help people transition negative thoughts into positive emotions. We will present a unique combination of cognitive restructuring, affirmation therapy, and logotherapy.

Cognitive restructuring is a very intriguing and powerful way to help people process or react to situations in a way that is helpful versus harmful. It is stated in one publication that, "Once our individual negative thought patterns are identified and examined, a technique called 'cognitive restructuring' helps us change the automatic way we think by finding positive, affirming approaches to life's ups and downs."[9] The automatic thoughts are very important because negative or positive emotions are stimulated from that point. It is so common for a cancer patient to automatically tie every event to the disease. If they feel stiff in their muscles or if they start with a little cough, instantly they think, "Maybe the cancer has spread or maybe it is growing." The reality is that stiff muscles and coughs are everyday occurrences for humans and they are probably not linked to cancer. But if a person's automatic thought is that every physical discomfort means that they are losing the battle to cancer, it will be very difficult for them to do away with immune depressing emotions.

I believe that we can show a patient how to reprogram the way he perceives and processes information about his illness through cognitive restructuring and affirmation therapy. I also believe that through these techniques, a patient can burn new neuron chains to replace previous negative thought patterns resulting in immunization from future stimulation of negative emotions.

Affirmation therapy will be a vital part of our program because so many people face an identity crisis upon receiving a cancer diagnosis. No matter whether a person is a top politician or a friendly person that works at the local library, their whole life and existence is reduced to the wrong identity. They are now cancer patients and nothing more. All else is lost. It is common for people to feel this way, but a person is never a disease. Life should not be put on hold. No one should ask permission from cancer to enjoy life. Life is to be lived regardless. Cancer must be put into the right perspective.

It is such a wonderful thing to see people rediscover themselves and realize that cancer is just a circumstance and it does not define who they are. Affirmation therapy is an effective way of helping people find value. By affirming a person, they can begin to realize that even in difficult circumstances, they can have meaning and can share meaningful moments with others. They can have a positive influence in other's lives.

One of the most meaningful experiences that takes place at Oasis of Hope is the forming of friendships between patients. To see one patient forget about his own condition to focus to the needs of another patient is moving. When this happens, it becomes apparent that the patient has discovered himself again. In fact, there are times when a patient discovers himself for the first time through the experience of cancer.

Life becomes invaluable when it is meaningful. The whole point of cognitive restructuring is to do away with negative automatic thoughts that depress the person physically, emotionally and spiritually and replace them with uplifting cognitions that open them up to meaningful experiences. Then, affirmation therapy emphasizes the significant and positive attributes of a person that make life meaningful. Cancer is temporary. But meaning is everlasting.

For long-term success, patients will be introduced to logotherapy. Viktor Frankl, the pysichiatrist who invented logotherapy, eloquently explains the direct link between life and meaning in his landmark book *Man's Search For Meaning*. He also explains the link between hope and life.[10] I propose that if a person does not sense meaning in his life, he will not find the will to live. Even if we accomplish improvements through cognitive restructuring and affirmation therapy, a person must find a reason to live or the results will be temporary.

In the next chapter, I will share with you from my heart about where many of my patients have found meaning. I too have found meaning for life in this world through a spiritual understanding.

# CHAPTER FOURTEEN

## Learning New Tricks

Children are like sponges. They can learn anything...and quickly. I'm convinced now that if you place a child in a room full of random gears, transistors, etcetera, you can come back in an hour and the child will have assembled a fully functioning combustion engine. A child's capacity to absorb new information and assimilate it into everyday life is truly amazing.

Take a small boy, for example. By age three, a small boy's brain will develop an area known to medical professionals as the "tape recorder." This area of the brain enables the boy to memorize just about anything and use it in context. This can lead to some very embarrassing moments.

One time, my nephew and his family were visiting a new church and after the service they walked out into the foyer where the pastor was greeting people. The pastor leaned down to my nephew's young son Joshua and asked, "How are you today, young man?"

"I'm five-years-old today," Joshua replied.

"My goodness," said the pastor, his eyes widening, "You're getting old!"

"I'm not old," Joshua answered, "When you get old, your butt gets big and jiggly." My nephew still wears a paper bag over his head.

While children have the capacity to learn just about anything, including extremely difficult subjects like nuclear physics and macramé, adults seem to have lost some of this ability. Just sit a technologically illiterate adult down in front of a computer and this point will become amply clear to you. After he breaks the CD tray, by using it as a cup holder, and kicks the tower when you suggest he "boot up," you will realize you're engaged in a pointless exercise.

I remember the story a teacher told me about the time his school got a state-of-the-art copy machine in the staff workroom. He was preparing some materials one morning when he heard someone muttering behind him. He turned around and there was this veteran teacher hunched over the machine. "What's wrong Judy?" he asked walking over to help.

"This stupid thing won't work right," she grumbled.

My teacher friend looked at the machine and then noticed that someone had left a book in the document feed tray on the side. "Here's your problem," he said, "Someone left a book in the feeder tray."

"I did," she frowned, "I'm trying to copy chapter seventeen, but it's not working." It did not take a tremendous amount of effort on my friend's part to help Judy out that morning.

While we can laugh at stories like these, there is a hard truth here when it comes to dismantling cancer. It is critical that the cancer patient learn a host of things in order to alter lifestyle in healthy ways. It is unreasonable to expect to have victory over cancer without eliminating the very things that make us susceptible to the disease. There are three areas of lifestyle that must be altered: environment, diet, and activity.

I'm not sure the average person realizes just how toxic the environment can be. There are many things around us that can create toxic stress in our bodies. Sometimes these things are obvious. If you are a lung cancer survivor and you live in a home where three people smoke cigarettes, you *know* something has to change. But do you know that the residual fumes from toxic house cleaners can have the same effect? Do you know how many toxins find their way into the water that comes from your tap? Do you know how many toxins are belched into the air and make it through the inadequate filtration system that comes standard on most home air/heating units?

The good news is that there are some simple and easy ways to eliminate toxins from our everyday environment. At Oasis, we are committed to teaching our patients how to do that.

Another source of toxins is the food in our diet. The chemicals used to process many popular foods items can place incredible amounts of toxic stress upon the body. The good news is that these chemicals are not the source of flavor in these foods. Eliminating the use of processed foods does not mean eliminating flavor from the diet. It is true that non-processed foods are often more expensive, but if the cost of saving a few bucks is cancer, it's worth it to pay the extra money for healthy non-toxic food. It is also true that non-processed foods are prone to spoil faster, but it really isn't that hard to buy smaller amounts of food and double the trips to the grocery store. It is important to teach patients which foods to avoid as they walk the aisles of the grocery store.

While eliminating toxic products from the diet is important, it is equally important to add foods that equip the body with the tools it needs to prevent disease. There are many foods that contain powerful disease preventative substances. Again, these are normal, tasty foods like tomatoes, red grapes, garlic, and olive oil. At Oasis, we have cooking classes to help patients learn how to incorporate many of these "super-foods" into their diet.

Finally, the types of activities we engage in can be an incredible source of stress. This is the most difficult aspect of lifestyle to alter. Many people live incredibly busy lives and are used to functioning for prolonged periods of time under intense stress. They don't live in a balanced state and fail to relax and exercise. This kind of activity can severely depress the immune system, making a person much more susceptible to disease.

It is important to talk candidly with cancer patients about scaling back or eliminating the activities that cause stress and unrest. Among other things, our physical therapist teaches patients how to breathe better to increase oxygenation, perform mild exercises to gently increase circulation and metabolic function. Learning activities that encourage the release of stress is a huge part of disease management and prevention.

Again, this is a treatment component that is sorely lacking in the vast majority of cancer centers around the world, but not at Oasis. Our education program is comprehensive and we encourage both the patient and her companion to attend every session. In this way, the patient doesn't have to make the changes alone and the companion derives a benefit, as well. Finally, we prescribe a five-year follow up program, to encourage patients to make the changes for life.

It is so important to alter lifestyle in healthy ways. To continue doing the same old things and expect different results is the epitome of insanity. If people can learn to make common sense changes in their environment, diet, and activities, I know that their chances of remission will increase dramatically and their chances of getting a degenerative disease like cancer again will virtually disappear.

# CHAPTER FIFTEEN

## *True Spirit*

Maybe it's just me, but I get choked up when I feel blessed. It happened to me just the other night at the dinner table. My girls were home and my wife and I sat at the dinner table with my five children. It was kind of wet and drizzly outside, but the house was warm and cozy. Conversation was "ping-ponging" around the table and I had a moment. I sort of disappeared. I leaned back a little, everybody forgot about me for a second, and I just got to watch. My daughters and son laughed and their hands flew as they related some story to my wife, who laughed with them. My youngest watched them intently, his big eyes soaking in everything. I sat, tears rolling down my face, thinking to myself, "My God! Why me? What have I done to deserve this family? What a blessing they are to me."

Think over the last year. Do you remember any blessings you received? Maybe you got an unexpected check in the mail, maybe someone had an exceptionally kind thing to say to you, maybe you spent an amazing afternoon with your child, maybe you just stared into a spectacular sunset...or maybe...maybe you were diagnosed with cancer.

I know what you're thinking...and no, it isn't a typing error. I know when a person sits down with a doctor and hears the awful word "cancer," they don't jump out of the chair and shout, "Yes! What a blessing!" If they did, I would be a little concerned about them. Reacting to the news with shock, denial, fear, and grief is the much more "normal" response of the average person.

Yet, there comes a point in the battle with cancer that I mentioned in chapter twelve. There comes a point when the patient asks the same question I asked that night at the dinner table with my family. They ask, "My God! Why me?" I believe with every fiber of my being that the answer to that question is the key to victory over cancer and everything else life can throw at us.

There is a poster in just about every self-respecting bible bookstore in the world that lists the names of Christ. He is called the Almighty, the Bread of Life, the Creator, the First and Last, the Good Shepherd, the Holy One, the King of Kings, the Lamb of God, the Messiah, the Prince of Peace, the Redeemer, the Savior, the Truth, and the Word...just to name a few. The list of names is very long, but nowhere in it will you find the name rescuer. It is not there. Savior is there, but the two do not mean exactly the same thing.

While it is true that the definitions are almost identical, both words meaning one who delivers someone from destruction or danger, believers understand that the name Savior is a reference to God's plan to save us from the eternal destruction brought about by sin. Modern day psychologists have altered the meaning of the word rescuer somewhat. Today, rescuer can often refer to someone who bails others out of difficult circumstances. Often the connotation is negative.

I believe the name rescuer is not found in that list because the name Redeemer is there instead. A redeemer is not a rescuer. A redeemer does not bail others out of difficult circumstances. A redeemer is a person who restores things to their rightful place. Christ is the Redeemer.

Let me tell you the rightful place for every event and moment that transpires here on earth. "We know that in *all things* God works for the good of those who love him." The quote is from Romans 8:28 in the New Testament *(New International Version)*. This means Christ's job as the Redeemer is to take every situation that life throws at you and use it so that it brings you a blessing...even cancer.

It doesn't mean that we will understand the blessing right away. It doesn't mean that we're wrong or weak for feeling shock, denial, fear, and anger. What this means is that God is good...always. What this means is that when life asks us to walk a rough road, there is a Redeemer who walks every single inch of it with us, who comforts us as we walk it, and who transforms the journey into a blessing, no matter where it leads. Let me clarify this. Cancer is not a blessing, but if looked for new blessings will be found through the difficult challenge that otherwise would have never been experienced.

The glaring weak point of virtually every cancer clinic in the world is the failure to recognize the importance of encouraging the patient to walk the rough road *with* the Redeemer. I believe that nothing we do at Oasis is more important than that. In fact, if I had to reduce the treatment program to a single therapy...this would be it. I am convinced that nothing we do here impacts the lives of patients more than prayer and devotions.

Besides the obvious spiritual benefit, clinical trials indicate that there is healing power in prayer.[1] Some people believe that there is no power inherent in the discipline itself, but science proves that belief to be misguided. There is a natural therapeutic effect in prayer that benefits a patient. Beyond that, prayer is a way to connect to a God who possesses unlimited healing resources. It would be foolish not to encourage every patient to pray regularly.

Devoting time to reading God's word is an integral part of the Oasis treatment program. Every morning, a pastor or missionary leads patients in biblical devotions. Hearing about God's love and God's promises builds faith and promotes peace. Patients tell me that spending time in God's word helps them to be much more positive about the challenges they face. God's word is the source of life.

We also seek to encourage every member of our staff to live by God's principals, particularly in their interactions with our patients. We want our patients to be showered with love and care on each and every visit. When people are diagnosed with cancer, they are all too ready to assume the identity of a cancer patient. We encourage all of our staff to share healing words with patients, to help patients rebuild their self-esteem, and to strengthen the faith of our patients. Proverbs 18:21 tells us that death and life are on the tongue. We choose to speak life into our patients and one another. That is the true spirit lived out every day at the Oasis of Hope.

# CHAPTER SIXTEEN

## *Great Expectations*

The first time I went roller skating was with the church youth group as a young teenager. There was a girl in the group that I was eager to impress so, naturally, I was totally convinced that something disastrous was going to happen. The closest I had gotten to roller skating before that fateful day was the time the sister of a neighborhood friend left one of her skates at the foot of the stairs in her house. We tumbled down the stairs toward the kitchen and I planted my foot right on the skate. I'm sure I earned my pilot's wings that day, because I took off and it felt like hours before I hit the ground.

Needless to say, the experience made an unpleasant impression on me and filled me with the desire to throttle the idiot who first got the idea of attaching wheels to the bottom of a pair of shoes. So, I was less than enthusiastic about this particular church outing.

We arrived at the roller rink and I immediately broke into a sweat. I wanted this girl to think I was cool. I didn't want her to watch me use my head like a battering ram. My "friends," and I use that term loosely, assured me that everything would be fine and that I would catch on to this roller skating thing in no time at all.

I went and rented a pair of skates, which were the color of baby puke, and strapped them to my feet. I moved to the opening to the rink where scores of young boys and girls now swirled gracefully in a perpetual left-hand turn. I took a few tentative steps and...I was off. I was not the picture of perfection by any stretch of the imagination, but I was actually managing to look coordinated. Then, I saw her.

She was at the wall about twenty yards up and looking my direction. I thought, "Don't fall, don't fall, don't fall." So, of course, I fell. I'm not even sure what happened to tell you the truth, but I'm confident that my body did things that are not humanly possible. I'm positive that the contortionists from the *Cirque du Soliel* would have been proud, and that there is probably a very humorous dance named after me somewhere.

You are probably familiar with the concept of self-fulfilling prophecy. It is the irony that what one worries could happen does happen because anxiety makes it happen. While self-fulfilling prophecy can be disastrous, as it was for me on that day, it can also be a blessing. What a person hopes will happen can happen because faith will make it happen.

Many people consider the body to be the primary battleground for cancer but I believe the real war is fought in the heart and mind of the patient. The fear of cancer causes a person to believe that he will die, and if he is fully convinced of his imminent demise, the likelihood of survival is miniscule. Negative emotions actually have a devastating physiological impact.

Yet, if a patient is freed of the fear, healing becomes much more likely. That freedom also opens the door to other meaningful experiences that are not affected by the advance or remission of the cancer. The person who experiences that freedom is victorious no matter what the lab results are. I want to share with you the stories of three cancer victors. Two are still living, one has passed away, but all three defeated cancer. The words in quotations were spoken or written by the patient.

## Dee

"Twelve years ago I was diagnosed with breast cancer. I was devastated and shocked. First of all, I couldn't believe this could happen to me. I had never been sick, not even with a cold, and I had always considered myself to be a very healthy person. Immediately, I had a decision to make—*Did I want to live or did I want to die?* My choice was obvious.

Coming home from the hospital, I knew I must take charge of my life. I had just gone through an eight-hour modified radical mastectomy, and with my determination to survive, my journey began.

Fortunately, the first part of my journey took me to Oasis of Hope Hospital where I met and became a patient of Dr. Francisco Contreras. Immediately, my life was touched in a positive way by a staff and an environment that reassured and comforted me. They offered me peace and healing. I was treated in not only a professional way, but as a personal family member.

Oasis' focus was on the whole patient, not just the disease. With the assistance of Dr. Contreras and the hospital staff, I learned how to take charge of my life. This was the real journey, the journey to healing. I soon became an avid student of nutrition and quickly learned how to apply the best of science and the best of nature to my personal life. I also learned health is the most valuable possession in life.

Cancer is the ultimate battle. It forces you to fight for your life. Cancer does not discriminate. Only a few years ago, cancer was referred to as a condition too awful to discuss. However, knowledge is a powerful weapon in the battle against cancer. Survivors know cancer can be conquered, and they learn to speak the language of warfare. They truly have fought an enemy within—not simply the intruding cells, but denial, anger, and despair, as well.

Many cancer survivors consider the disease to have been a gift in a horrible package, a message too dire to ignore: life, which is indeed fleeting and precious, is a miracle and a gift from God. I know hope is the most powerful medicine of all. Illness is an opportunity for growth, and the healing part comes from the ability to deal with whatever illness is troubling you. It's all about finding peace of mind.

How did an experience so tragic bring good into my life? It was a lesson to teach me where to turn to in a crisis. It pulled me into a dark valley, dropping me along the way—forcing me to rest and learn to trust. Psalm 46:10 says, 'Be still and know that I am God.'

He was in control. I emerged on the mountaintop, in the same world but with a different appreciation of life and a closer relationship with my Savior. Yes, I touched the rose and felt the thorn. I've seen my life go from 'vision to victory.'

We cannot tell what may happen to us in the strange medley of life, but we can decide what happens within us...how we take it and what we do with it. That's what really counts in the end—how to take the raw stuff of life and make it a thing of worth and beauty. That is the test of living. The magic of life can never end, for it's filled with all life's greatest gifts—our family and friends.

If you are struggling with illness, remember the importance of a positive mental attitude and do not give up hope. Arm yourself with knowledge about your illness, and become an active participant in your treatment plans."

## Jack

Jack Riley was a senior triathlete. He entered races that involved three phases—swimming, biking, and running. A grueling sport even for the young, Jack had begun running triathlons later in life. A former drinker, smoker, and junk food advocate, Jack had traded in his bourbon glass for running shoes in mid-life. Jack competed in 644 marathons and triathlons.

After being diagnosed and treated for prostate cancer, Jack, a thirty-year resident of Alamo, California, became a community hero in 1996 when he was elected to carry the Olympic Torch in San Francisco during the torch relay. He passed the flame on to the next runner, dipped his foot in the Pacific Ocean, then ran, biked, and swam 3,300 miles to the Olympic stadium in Atlanta, his personal Olympic torch in hand. He continued on until he arrived at the Atlantic Ocean.

In 1997 he ran, biked, and swam 1,700 miles from Vancouver, Canada, to Tijuana, Mexico. Jack's runs took him through three hundred towns. Through the media, over fifteen million people were made aware of his quest. For Jack, the highlight of his trips was visiting children's cancer centers in the major cities and helping to cheer up those children and give them courage to fight their battle against cancer.

In the last phase of his life, Jack wasn't dwelling on dying; he was concentrating on living. When I asked Jack what the motivation was for his transnational triathalons, he replied, "I am a competitor. I guess it is just in my blood. If I can do this for a good cause...well, that's what life is all about. I will do this as long as I can...as long as God gives me the physical, mental, and emotional ability. I see cancer as a competitor, but I don't dwell on the other competitors. I dwell on my *own* performance, which is in the hands of God."

On Jack's third and final triathlon of hope, he made it from the Pacific Ocean through thirteen cities in California and Arizona. At New Mexico's border, his body gave out, though his spirit never did. Jack Riley passed away on July 1, 1998. His wife told me that he died the way he wanted to die, serving others and fighting for a cure to cancer.

Jack Riley was, and continues to be, a role model for those with a cancer challenge because he kept a positive attitude. In a day when it is difficult to find a hero, Jack is one of mine because he had courage, commitment, love, integrity, and focus. Jack was a friend whose memory motivates me to do something meaningful with my life. When I feel challenged and even overwhelmed by the tasks of a day, I think of Jack. He had cancer, and yet he crossed the United States more than two times on his own power.

*William*

One day at the hospital, we were having a prayer service. One of our pastors approached a patient named William who was there on a follow-up visit. When William was asked if he wanted prayer for healing he responded, "I don't need to be healed of cancer. I have already been blessed more than I deserve. I have been married to my lovely wife for fifty years and some wonderful things have come

125

about since I was diagnosed with cancer. A number of my friends who didn't know Christ now do because they started to spend more time with me and we would pray together. Also, I have three children, all of whom had broken marriages. The kids started to get together to pray and now two of those marriages have been restored and I am waiting for the third one to get back together with his wife. Now do you understand why I am not worried about the cancer?"

Many people feel that anything less than a cure is a failure when it comes to cancer. My patients have demonstrated to me just how incorrect that point of view is. I encourage my patients to search for meaning through the experience and look for the hidden miracles in the process. That is what William did. I also ask people to expand their definition of what a valid outcome looks like.

For many patients, the valid outcome is the enjoyment of many years of quality living even though the cancer persists. I will never forget the time I accompanied my father to the famed Sloan-Kettering cancer center in New York to share successful case studies with some of the leading oncologists in the world. My father put up a patient's diagnostic chest x-ray alongside a post treatment x-ray. The tumor was still there. One of the oncologists stood up and stated, "That's not a successful case."

He left the room and returned with comparative x-rays of one of his patients. The diagnostic x-ray showed a tumor and the posttreatment x-ray did not. My father congratulated the doctor and asked how the patient was doing. The oncologist stated with no remorse, "The patient died, but the treatment was successful."

My father humbly pointed out that even though cancer was still present in the patient of the case he presented, the x-rays were taken ten years apart and the patient continued to live and work with the cancer completely under control. I was dumbfounded when the oncologists told my father that it was a nice story but that only objective results, such as measurable tumor reduction, constituted a valid outcome. The patients who have found a way to peacefully co-exist with a cancer would disagree. Controlling cancer is also a valid outcome.

For some patients, a valid outcome is outliving their prognosis by months and sometimes even years. This outcome is truly a success when patients really begin to *live*. Patch Adams once told me, "I know we have a world panic about cancer. But the worst cancer is being alive and not enjoying it, not feeling gratitude, not loving, not living. It is not the dying of death that is really the big deal; it is the dying in life that is bad. To go around thinking, 'Life is a struggle, life is terrible and then you die,' that's the worst cancer. Being in this miracle of life and throwing it away is much worse. The hope with cancer is not whether we are going to get rid of it. We are never going to end death. We want to have a little more life so we may experience the living that we have been hoping for in the future, when, in fact, anyone can have it today."

I often ask patients, "What will you do differently if you are cured of cancer?" When they tell me their answer, I suggest that they begin living their dreams today instead of waiting. If your life is to be extended, make it count. And if you live life to the fullest, every extra day becomes a day to celebrate.

It is always wonderful to see people come to terms with life and the people around them. My father received a letter from a woman telling him that her husband had passed away but that she had much to be grateful for. While he was being treated, he found peace and love and was able to forgive his father for childhood abuse. After that, he lived six more months and his wife said that he was a new man. He had never been affectionate with his children but in those six months, his girls experienced what it was to have a loving father. The man was not cured, he did not co-exist for long with the cancer, but, he experienced life with his family that they might not have otherwise had.

You can kick the feet out from under cancer if you can adapt great expectations. If a cure is the only acceptable resolution for you, you just might miss out on the incredible blessing that God has for you.

# CHAPTER SEVENTEEN

## *Take Charge*

If you are a cancer patient, whether or not you are considering coming to the Oasis of Hope, I would encourage you to adopt these recommendations. They have helped patients experience victory over cancer.

First, prepare your mind for success. Be at peace with your choice of therapy. Even though wisdom is in the multitude of opinions, at the end of the day you must make your choice having weighed all options. Nine out of ten times, people will voice disapproval to your decision. They'll say chemotherapy is toxic, alternative therapy is...well, alternative. Once all the cards are on the table let your gut or, better yet, your God guide your decision. Remember that nothing is written in stone. You can change your mind at any time. To every therapy you can say yes, no, maybe, or not yet. Your needs are the ones that have to be met not everybody else's.

Second, accept the doctor's prognosis as a professional opinion; not God's truth. Most people are easily persuaded by an authority figure. Doctors are trained to give a statistical estimation of your personal condition. Remember, it's only an estimate. If your doctor has sentenced you to death and attached a timetable to the rest of your life, you must process that prognosis with caution. Your doctor may be a medical authority figure, but he is not a prophet. Yes, statistics can be reliable sources of information but it is you who decides which group you want to identify with, the 70 percent chance group or the 30 percent chance group? Will Rogers said, "Most people are about as happy as they make up their minds to be." Never give up hope.

Third, prepare your body for success. Be diligent in your journey towards healing. Once you have chosen the therapy that's best for you, change any area of your lifestyle that could compromise the results. Make a commitment to stop smoking, drinking and eating junk food. Start exercising more, drinking water more, resting more, and *living* more.

Fourth, eat foods that promote health. There is no controversy over the connection between diet and health. Start consuming organic vegetables and fruits on a daily basis. If you insist on eating meats, eat them in moderation and make sure it is free range, free of hormones and antibodies. Avoid dairy products as much as possible. Stay away from any type of processed food, especially fast foods

Fifth, start supplementing your diet with vitamins, minerals, phytochemicals, enzymes, and amino acids. These are important resources that will enable your immune system to work better for you, some of them are even mild antitumor agents that will complement your therapy, be it alternative or orthodox.

Sixth, prepare your soul for success. Many of us rarely consider our spiritual status until we are faced with a crisis. The Chinese do not have a character for crisis; instead, they depict crisis by combining the character for danger with the one for opportunity. If you acknowledge that cancer not only presents a danger but an opportunity as well, you will be better equipped to come out on top. Patients who are able to put cancer in the "back seat" can go on with their lives without allowing the presence of a malignancy to consume them with fear.

Seventh, remember that God is in charge. Regardless of your personal beliefs, even if you are an agnostic, you recognize that a force greater than ours is at work in the universe. Some call it chance, but I like to call it God. If you allow God to help in your time of greatest need, I believe you will be spiritually healed, as well. Statistics show that spiritual fortitude helps cancer patients fare better.

# EPILOGUE

Friedrich Nietzsche said that a liar lies to others and that an optimist lies to himself. In the search for a cancer cure, many promises have come and gone and optimistic new promises are now viewed with skepticism. That is why receiving a diagnosis of cancer is so devastating; because one assumes that the odds of beating it are so infinitesimally small that it would be a waste of time trying. Patients often feel dead even though they are still walking among the living.

I choose to run counter to the current stream of thought. I agree that research should be objective and that we should be grounded in the real world. However, I'm optimistic that we can help cancer patients even more than we do today if we change our scientific paradigm.

The aim of mainstream medicine has been to destroy tumors through surgery, radiation, and chemotherapy. Incredibly, the medical community has been pursuing the same therapies, aided by new technology, expecting to obtain different results. Where is the logic in that?

There are new therapies like the human genome project that are rapidly changing the perspective of many doctors. In the near future, we may be able to target the cancer genes themselves or the proteins they produce. One such approach is Glevec, the first drug approved by the FDA for the treatment of cancer that is not chemotherapeutic. Glevec is in a new class of cancer drug and represents a shift in the scientific paradigm. This drug attacks proteins that help the cancer survive. Most therapies lack specificity, and kill normal cells as well as cancer cells.

For forty years we have treated patients with a completely different approach. At the Oasis of Hope the aim of treatment is not to destroy the tumor. Don't get me wrong, tumors are on our most wanted list, but they don't occupy the number one spot. But we look beyond tumor destruction to the restoration of natural defenses, avoidance of stressors, development of a healthy lifestyle, and spiritual/emotional support. Without a multi-faceted approach, no amount of chemotherapy or radiation will help.

In reflection at this four-decade milestone of cancer treatment at the Oasis of Hope, I would like to share the vision of what our organization will be doing over the next ten years. The list is a starting point because things are being discovered on a daily basis. I am sure that we will readjust this list numerous times. Nonetheless, here is a draft:

- Further develop the use of amygdalin as a prodrug
- Develop transimmunization
- Advance the use of Ozone and UV light
- Complete the design of a healing environment at the Oasis of Hope Hospital through electromagnetic field organizers, and air and water ionizers
- Help people create healing environments in their homes. This information will be available at *www.inhomeoasis.com*
- Open outpatient clinics in London, Seoul and other leading medical cities to increase influence and broaden our research base
- Integrate mind/spirit therapies into medical program and help patients structure themselves for success
- Increase commitment to educating the world on cancer prevention and treatment

The future of cancer therapy is a bright one if physicians will open their minds to an integrative and eclectic approach and stop searching for the cure. Medical pride means nothing to a patient in need.

On a final note, I wish to acknowledge that many people have worked to bring our message or a similar message to the general public. I cannot mention everyone but I would like to note a few people and organizations that have been important to increasing the consciousness of people to a different approach to cancer treatment. We have had strategic partners who have increased our ability to communicate our message worldwide including MN Japan, Wing Company, Inc., Amino Up Chemical Co., Ltd., Mr. Andrew Nuttall, and Mr. Chris Byrne, hundreds of people in Christian Broadcasting, Strang Communications, Authentic Media, Editrice IL DONO, Dr. Rhee, Peter Graham, and The Full Gospel Businessmen's Fellowship International. I also wish to recognize the tireless work of people and organizations like Edward Griffin, Phillip Day, Cancer Victors and Friends, the Issels Foundation, Burton Goldberg, the Cancer Control Society, the Cancer Aid & Research Fund, the National Health Federation, Dr. Patch Adams, and the Gerson Institute. I also thank all of the doctors and clinics that have incorporated our philosophy and protocols into their work. My father's deepest wish was to share what he learned with the world.

**Francisco Contreras, MD**

# Appendix I

## New Approach: Amygdalin as Tumoral Sensitizer (pro-drug) in the Induction of Apoptosis, via Reduction of Intracellular Cysteine Levels

Cancer cells have higher concentrations of cysteine and glutathione than healthy cells do. Glutathione makes tumors resistant to treatment. Amygdalin's cyanide lowers the levels of cysteine, which in turn lowers the concentrations of intracellular glutathione. Tumors with low concentrations of glutathione are sensitive to antitumor agents.

When amygdalin is taken, the body metabolizes it and cyanhydric acid (HCN) is produced.[1]   HCN, though highly toxic, is immediately converted into a non-toxic substance called thyocyanate (SCN). SCN consumes cysteine in an intracellular process. It is this function that makes amygdalin so vital in the treatment of cancer.[2]   The process is carried out by sulfur transferase enzymes, such as rhodenase, among others.[3] These enzymes contain an active site of cysteine (Cys), where the reaction that transforms cyanhydric acid into thyocyanate (HCN→SCN) takes place.[4]

This mediated function through sulfurtranferases depends on the intracellular level of cysteine[5] as the fundamental donor of the sulfur that is transferred in the reaction HCN→SCN. The strategic value in reducing cysteine levels in tumors has been well-documented by several researchers.[6]   One of the most important effects is the depletion of intracellular glutathione (GSH) whose concentration depends on the availability of cysteine.[7]   When concentrations of glutathione are low, apoptosis (programmed cell death) of tumor cells is promoted via the destabilization of mitochondrial membrane permeability.[8] In contrast, a high concentration of intracellular glutathione in tumors is related to the phenomena of Multi Drugs Resistant Tumor.[9] Furthermore, high levels of intracellular glutathione are responsible for the resistance tumors have to oxidative stress. This means that the tumors become resistant to radiation, chemotherapy, drugs, phytochemicals, or oxidative therapies.[10]

Lowering cysteine levels results in sensitization of tumors. This provides a tremendous advantage in the fight against cancer that should not be discarded by mainstream oncologists.[11] I predict that sensitizing malignant cells to oxidative stress will become the cutting edge of anticancer research. In our effort to find substances with these sensitizing properties, we continuously study compounds, especially those found in nature, which may aid antineoplastic treatments. Amygdalin can increase sensitization of certain tumors especially in combination with other substances such as vitamin C, theanine, vitamin K-3, arsenic trioxide (Aas2 O3), menadione and other substances that modulate glutathione and cysteine levels.[12]

# APPENDIX II

## Krebs' hypothesis: Amygdalin's mechanism of action

The highly toxic substance cyanhydric acid (HCN) is one of the end products of the hydrolysis of amygdalin. In order to produce it, ß-glucosidase is required. Rhodanese is an enzyme that performs a function of converting HCN to thyocyanate (SCN), a harmless substance. Rhodanese is part of the normal detoxification process of the body. However, in contrast with normal cells, cancerous cells are high in ß-glucosidase and low in rhodanese. Thus the normal cellular protective mechanism is decreased in tumor cells and they become more sensitive to the effects of the HCN, which depresses the enzyme functions of the cancer cell and thereby destroys it. Then, according to Ernest Krebs hypothesis, amygdalin's toxic effects are against the cancerous cell and not the host. [13]

# REFERENCES

*Chapter 1  Cancer Mythology*
1. Maxwell, John. Retrieved from Internet, April 15, 2004.
   http://www.quotationspage.com/search.php3?homesearch=john+
   maxwell&x=34&y=10

*Chapter 2  A Need For Change*
1. "The National Cancer Act of 1971". http://www3.cancer.gov/legis/
   1971canc.html
2. In 1889, Halsted described a radical operation of breast cancer.
   http://www.medicalarchives.jhmi.edu/halsted/haccomp.htm
3. American Cancer Society. The History of Cancer.
   http://www.cancer.org/docroot/CRI/content/CRI_2_6x_
   the_history_of_cancer_72.asp
4. See Anne MacLennan " No Advantage in Radical Over Total Mastectomy: 25-year Study"http://www.docguide.com/news/
   content.nsf/news/8525697700573E1885256C1D000E2E2A
   Bernard F, Jeong J, Anderson S et al. Twenty-five-year follow-up
   of a randomized trial comparing radical mastectomy, total mastectomy, and total mastectomy followed by irradiation. N Engl J Med
   2002;347:567-575.
   Veronesi U, Cascinelli N, Mariani L et al. Twenty-year follow-up of
   a randomized study comparing breast-conserving surgery with radical
   mastectomy for early breast cancer. N Engl J Med
   2002;347(16):1227-32.
5. See Moss, Ralph W. Chemo's Berlin Wall Crumbles.  The Cancer
   Chronicles. No. 7, December 1990.
   http://www.ralphmoss.com/ChemoBerlin.html
6. Bailar 3rd, JC and Elaine M. Smith. Progress against cancer? N Eng
   J Med 1986;314(19):1226-1232.
   Bailar 3rd, JC and Heather L. Gornik. Cancer undefeated. N Eng J
   Med 1997; 336(22):1569-1574.

## Chapter 7 Cleaning House

1. Olszewer E and Carter JP. EDTA Chelation in chronic degenerative disease. Med Hypotheses 1988;27:41-49.
2. Ibid.
3. Ibid.
4. Bosisio E, Benelli C and Pirola O. Effect of the flavonolignans of Silybum marianum L. on lipid peroxidation in rat liver microsomes and freshly isolated hepatocytes. Pharmacol Res 1992;25:147-154.
5. Saller R, Meier R and Brignoli R. The use of silymarin in the treatment of liver diseases. Drugs 2001;61(14):2035-2063.
6. Ibid.
7. Saller R, Meier R and Brignoli R. The use of silymarin in the treatment of liver diseases. Drugs 2001;61(14):2035-2063.
   Letteron P et al. Mechanism for the protective effects of silymarin against carbon tetrachloride-induced lipid peroxidation and hepatoxicity on mice. Biochem Pharmacol 1990;39:2027-2034.
   von Schonfeld J, Weisbrod B and Muller MK. Silibinin, a plant extract with antioxidant and membrane stabilizing properties, protects exocrine pancreas from cyclosporin A toxicity. Cell Mol Life Sci 1997; 53:917-920.
   Frederick H, et al. Silymarin—a phytopharmaceutical preparation for the treatment of toxic liver damage. Kassenmarzt 1990: 33:36-41.
   Valenzuela A et al. Silymarin protection against hepatic lipd peroxidation iduced by acute ethanol intoxication in the rat. Biochem Pharm 1985;34:2209-2212.
8. See note 5.
9. Wellington K and Jarvis B. Silymarin: a review of its clinical properties in the management of hepatic disorders. Bio Drugs 2001;15(7):465-489.
10. Panda K, Chattopadhyay R et al. Vitamin C prevents cigarette smoke-induced oxidative damage in vivo. Free Radic Biol Med 2000;29(2):115-124.
    Menzel DB. Antioxidant vitamins and prevention of lung disease. Ann NY Acad Sci 1992;669:141-155.
11. Schnare DW et al. Evaluation of a detoxification regimen for fat stored xenobiotics. Med Hypotheses 1982;9(3):265-282.
12. See note 10.

13. See note 11.

## Chapter 8 Nature's Pharmacy

1. Pinto JT, Qiao C, Xing J et al. Effects of garlic thioallyl derivatives on growth, glutathione concetration, and polyaminc formation of human prostate carcinoma cells in culture. Am J Clin Nutr 1997;66(2):398-405.
2. Takeyama H, Hoon DS, Saxton RE, Morton DL and Irie RF. Growth inhibition and modulation of cell markers of melanoma by S-allyl cysteine. Oncology 1993;50(1):63-69.
3. Welch C, Wuarin L and Sidell N. Antiproliferative effect of garlic compound S-allyl cysteine on human neuroblastoma cells in vitro. Cancer Lett 1992;63(3):211-219.
4. Ibid.
5. Li G, Qiao CH, Lin RI et al. Antiproliferative effects of garlic constituents on cultured human breast cancer cells. Oncol Rep 1995;2:787-791.
6. Sundaram SG and Millner JA. Diallyl disulfide suppresses the growth of human colon tumor cell xenografts in athymic nude mice. J Nutr 1996;126(5):1355-1361.
7. Wargovich MJ, Woods C, Eng VW et al. Chemoprevention of N-nitrosomethylbenzylamine-induced esophageal cancer in rats by the naturally occurring thioether, diallyl sulfide. Cancer Res 1988;48(23):6872-6875.
8. Wattenberg LW, Sparnins VL and Barany G. Inhibition of N-nitrosodiethylamine carcinogenesis in mice by naturally occurring organosulfur compounds and monoterpenes. Cancer Res 1989;49(10):2689-2692.
9. Sparnins Vl, Mott AW, Barany G and Wattenberg LW. Effects of allyl methyl trisulfide on glutathione S-transferease activity and BP-induced neoplasia in the mouse. Nutr Cancer 1986;8(3):211-215.
10. See note 5.
11. Nagourney RA. Garlic: Medicinal food or nutritious medicine. J Medicinal Food 1998;II(1):13-28.
12. Nagai K. Effect of garlic extract in prevention of virus infections. Kansenshigaku Zasshi 1973;47(4):111-115.
   Abdullah TH, Kandil O, Elkadi A et al. Garlic revisited: therapeutic for the major diseases of our time? J Natl Med Assoc 1988;80(4):439-445.

13. Nagourney RA. Garlic: Medicinal food or nutritious medicine. J Medicinal Food 1998;II(1):13-28.

   Moriguchi T, Saito H and Nishiyama N. Aged garlic extract prolongs longevity and improves spatial memory deficit in senescence-accelerated mouse. Biol Pharm Bull 1996;19(2):305-307.

   Moriguchi T, Saito H and Nishiyama N. Anti-aging effect of aged garlic extract in the inbread brain atrophy mouse model. Clin Experimen Pharmacol Physiol 1997; 24:235-242.

14. Steiner M, Khan AH, Holbert D and I-San Lin R. A double-blind crossover study in moderately hypercholesterolemic men that compared the effect of aged garlic extract and placebo administration on blood lipids. Am J Clin Nutr 1996; 64:866-870.

   Lau BH. Supression of LDL oxidation by garlic. J Nutr 2001;131(3S):985S-988S.

15. Morioka N, Sze LL, Morton DL and Irie RF. A protein fraction from aged garlic extract enhances cytotoxicity and proliferation of human lymphocytes mediated by interleukin-2 and concanavalin A. Cancer Immunol Immunother 1993;37(5):316-322.

16. Moriguchi T, Saito H and Nishiyama N. Aged garlic extract prolongs longevity and improves spatial memory deficit in senescence-accelerated mouse. Biol Pharm Bull 1996;19(2):305-307.

17. Moriguchi T, Saito H and Nishiyama N. Anti-aging effect of aged garlic extract in the inbread brain atrophy mouse model. Clin Experimen Pharmacol Physiol 1997; 24:235-242.

18. Giovanucci E. Tomatoes, tomato-based products, lycopene, and cancer: Review of the epidemiologic literature. J Natl Cancer Inst 1999; 91:317-331.

19. Agarwal S and Rao AV. Tomato lycopene and its role in human health and chronic disease. CMAJ 2000;163(6):739-744.

   Franceshi S, Bidoli E, La Vecchia C et al. Tomatoes and the risk of digestive-tract cancers. Int J Cancer 1994;59:181-184.

20. See note 18.

21. Greenlee RT, Murray T, Bolden S and Wingo PA. Cancer Statistics, 2000. CA Cancer J Clin 2000;50:7-33.

22. Giovannucci E. A review of epidemiologic studies of tomatoes, lycopene, and prostate cancer. Exp Biol Med 2002;227:852-859.

23. Lu Q-Y, Hung J-C, Heber D et al. Inverse associations between plasma lycopene and other carotenoids and prostate cancer. Cancer

Epidemiol Biomarkers Preven 2001;10:749-756.

24. Sauer LA, Dauchy RT and Blask DE. Polyunsaturated fatty acids, melatonin, and cancer. Biochem Pharmacol 2001; 61(12):1455-1462.

25. Lissoni P. Is there a role for melatonin in supportive care? Support Care Cancer 2002;10(2):110-116.

26. Ibid.

27. Ibid.

28. Ibid.

29. *Cachexia*: A profound and marked state of constitutional disorder; general ill health and malnutrition. [Dorland's Medical Illustrated Dictionary (*DMID*). Philadelphia:Saunders,1981.]

30. *Asthenia*: Lack or loss of strenght and energy; weakness. (*DMID*)

31. *Thrombocytopenia*: Decrease in the number of blood platelets. (*DMID*)

32. *Lymohocytopenia:* Reduction in the number of lymphocytes in the blood. (*DMID*)

33. See note 25.

34. Bubenik GA, Blask DE, Brown GM et al. Prospects of the clinical utilization of melatonin. Biol Signals Recep 1998; 7(4):195-219.

35. Meloni G, Vignetti M and Pogliani E. Interleukin-2 therapy in relapsed acute myclogcnous leukemia. Cancer J Sci Am 1997; 3 (Suppl 1): S43-S47.

36. Cos S and Sánchez-Barceló EJ. Melatonin, experimental basis for a possible application in breast cancer prevention and treatment. Histol Histopathol 2000;15:637-647.

37. Reiter RJ. Functional pleiotroy of the neurohormone melatonin: antioxidant protection and neuroendocrine regulation. Front Neuroendocrin 1995;16:383-415.
    Karbownik M and Reiter RJ. Antioxidative effects of melatonin in protection against cellular damage caused by ionizing radiation. Proc Soc Exp Biol Med 2000; 225(1):9-22.

38 Menendez-Pelaez A, Poeggeler B, Reiter RJ et al. Nuclear localization of melatonin in different mammalian tissues: immunocythochemical and radioimmunoassay evidence. J Cell Biochem 1993;53:372-382.

39. Frenkel K. Carcinogen mediated oxidant formation and oxidative DNA damage. Pharmacol Ther 1992; 53:127-166.

40. See note 36.

41. Karbownik M and Reiter RJ. Antioxidative effects of melatonin in protection against cellular damage caused by ionizing radiation. Proc Soc Exp Biol Med 2000; 225(1):9-22.

42. Burikhanov RB, Walkame K, Igarashi Y et al. Suppressive effect of active hexose correlated compound (AHCC) on thymic apoptosis induced by dexamethasone in the rat. Endocr Regul 2000;34(4):181-188.

43. Matsushita K, Kuramitsu Y, Ohiro Y et al. Combination therapy of active hexose correlated compound plus UFT significantly reduces the metastasis of rat mammary adenocarcinoma. Anticancer Drugs. 1998;9(4):343-350.

44 Ibid.

45. Aejmelaeus R, Mets-Ketel T, Laippala P et al. Ubiquinol-10 and total peroxyl radical trapping capacity of LDL lipoproteins during aging and the effects of Q10 supplementation. Mol Aspects Med 1997;18 (Suppl):S113-S120.

46. Kalen A, Appelkvist EL and Dallner G. Age-related changes in the lipid compositions of rat and human tissues. Lipids 1989; 24:579-581.

Kontush A, Reich A, Baum K et al. Plasma ubiquinol-10 is decreased in patients with hyperlipidaemia. Atheros 1997;129:119-126.

Folkers K, Littarru GP and Ho L. Evidence for a deficiency of coenzyme Q10 in human heart disease. Int J Vitamin Nutr Res 1970; 40:380-390.

47. Folkers K. Relevance of the biosynthesis of coenzyme Q10 and of the four bases of DNA as a rationale for the molecular causes of cancer and a therapy. Biochem Biophys Res Commun 1996;224:358-361.

Sinatra ST. "Care", cancer and coenzyme Q10. J Am Coll Cardiol 1999;33 (3):897-899.

48. Beyer RE. The participation of coenzyme Q10 in free radical production and antioxidation. Free Radic Biol Med 1990; 8:545-565.

Huertas JR, Martinez-Velasco E, Ibañez S et al. Virgin olive oil and coenzyme Q10 protect heart mitochondria from peroxidative damage during aging. Biofactors 1999; 9 (2-4):337-343.

49. Folkers K, Brown R, Judy WV and Morita M. Survival of cancer patients on therapy with Coenzyme Q10. Biochem Bipophys Res Commun 1993;192:241-245.

50. Ibid.
51. Lockwood K, Moesgaard S and Folkers K. Partial and complete regression of breast cancer in patients in relation to dosage of coenzyme Q10. Biochem Biophys Res Commun 1994; 199: 1504-1508.
52. Lockwood K, Moesgaard S, Yamamoto T and Folkers K. Progress on therapy of breast cancer with coenzyme Q10 and the regression of metastases. Biochem Biophys Res Commun 1995;212:172-177.
53. Ibid.
54. Stark AH and Mador Z. Olive oil as a functional food: epidemiology and nutritional approaches. Nutr Rev 2002;60(6):170-176.
    Visioli F and Galli C. Biological properties of olive oil phytochemicals. Crit Rev Food Sci Nutr 2002;42(3):209-221.
    Kushi L and Giovannucci E. Dietary fat and cancer. Am J Med 2002; 113 (Suppl 9 B):63S-70S.
55. Visioli F and Galli C. Biological properties of olive oil phytochemicals. Crit Rev Food Sci Nutr 2002;42(3):209-221.
    Visioli F, Bellomo G, Montedoro GF and Galli C. Low density lipoprotein oxidation is inhibited in vitro by olive oil constituents. Atheroesclerosis 1995;117:25-32.
56. Visioli F, Bellomo G and Galli C. Free radial-scavenging properties of olive oil polyphenols. Biochem Biophys Res Comm 1998;247:60-64.
57. Thuy NT, He P and Takeuchi H. Comparative effect of dietary olive, safflower, and linseed oils on spontaneous liver tumorigenesis in C3H/He mice. J Nutr Sci Vitaminol 2001;47(5):363-366.
58. Simopoulos AP. Evolutionary aspects of omega-3 fatty acid in the food supply. Prostanglandis Leukotrienes and Essential Fatty Acids. 1999;60(5-6):42-49.
59. Kris-Etherton PM, Taylor DS, Yu-Poth S et al. Polyunsaturated fatty acids in the food chain in the United States. Am J Clin Nutr 2000; 71 (Suppl):179S-188S.
60. Ibid.
61. Wagner VH et al. Chemistry and analysis of silymarin from Silybum marianum Gaertn. Arzneim-Forsch 1974;24:466-471.
62. Letteron P et al. Mechanism for the protective effects of silymarin against carbon tetrachloride-induced lipid peroxidation and hepatotoxicity in mice. Biochem Pharmacol 1990; 39:2027-2034.
63. Ahmad N et al. Skin cancer chemopreventive effects of a flavonoid

antioxidant silymarin are mediated via impairment of receptor tyrosine kinase signaling and perturbation in cell cycle progression. Biochem Biophys Res Commun 1998; 248:294-301.

Lahiri-Chattergee SK et al. A flavonoid antioxidant, silymarin, affords exceptionally high protection against tumor promotion in SENCAR mouse skin tumorigenesis model. Cancer Res 1999; 59:622-623.

Singh RP, Dhanalakshmi S et al. Dietary feeding of silibinin inhibits advance human prostate carcinoma growth in athymic nude mice and increases plasma insulin-like growth factor-binding protein -3 levels. Cancer Res 2002;62:3063-3069.

Tyagi A, Bhatia N, Condon MS et al. Antiproliferative and apoptotic effects on silibinin in rat prostate cancer cells. Prostate 2002;53;211-217.

Zi X et al. Anti-carcinogenic effect of a flavonoid antioxidant silymarin in human breast cancer cells MDA-MB 468: induction of G1 arrest through an increase in Cipl/p21 concomitant with a decrease in kinase activity of CDKs and associated cyclins. Clin Cancer Res 1998; 4:1055-1064.

Sharma G, Singh RP et al. Silibinin induces growth inhibition and apoptotic cell death in human lung carcinoma cells. Anticancer Res 2003;23(3B):2649-2655.

Yang Sh, Lin JK, Chen WS and Chiu JH. Anti-angiogenic effect of silymarin on colon cancer LoVo cell line. J Surg Res 2003;113(1);133-138.

Agarwal C, Singh RP et al. Silibinin upregulates the expression of cyclin-dependent kinase inhibitors and causes cell cycle arrest and apoptosis in human colon carcinoma HT-29 cells. Oncogene 2003;22(51):8271-8272.

Vinh PQ, Sugie S et al. Chemopreventive effects of a flavonoid antioxidant silymarin on N-butyl-N-(4-hydroxybutyl) nitrosamine-induced urinary bladder carcinogenesis in male ICR mice. Jpn J Cancer Res 2002;93:42-49.

64. Singh RP, Dhanalakshmi S et al. Dietary feeding of silibinin inhibits advance human prostate carcinoma growth in athymic nude mice and increases plasma insulin-like growth factor-binding protein -3 levels. Cancer Res 2002;62:3063-3069.

Singh RP, Tyagi AK, Zhao J and Agarwal R. Silymarin inhibits growth and causes regression of established skin tumors in SENCAR mice via modulation of nitrogen-activated protein kinase and induction of apoptosis. Carcinogenesis 2002;23(2);499-510.

65. Vinh PQ, Sugie S et al. Chemopreventive effects of a flavonoid antioxidant silymarin on N-butyl-N-(4-hydroxybutyl) nitrosamine-induced urinary bladder carcinogenesis in male ICR mice. Jpn J Cancer Res 2002;93:42-49.

66. Tyagi A, Bhatia N, Condon MS et al. Antiproliferative and apoptotic effects on silibinin in rat prostate cancer cells. Prostate 2002;53:211-217.

Agarwal C, Singh RP et al. Silibinin upregulates the expression of cyclin-dependent kinase inhibitors and causes cell cycle arrest and apoptosis in human colon carcinoma HT-29 cells. Oncogene 2003;22(51):8271-8272.

67. Agarwal C, Singh RP et al. Silibinin upregulates the expression of cyclin-dependent kinase inhibitors and causes cell cycle arrest and apoptosis in human colon carcinoma HT-29 cells. Oncogene 2003;22(51):8271-8272.

Zi X and Agarwal R. Silibinin decreases prostate-specific antigen with cell growth inhibition via G1 arrest, leading to differentiation of prostate carcinoma cells: Implications for prostate cancer intervention. Proc Natl Acad Sci. USA 1999; 96:7490-7495.

*Chapter 9  A Combined Effort*

1. See Table 1, Chapter 3.

2. Moertel CG, Fleming TR, Rubin J et al. A clinical trial of amygdalin (Laetrile) in the treatment of human cancer. N Eng J Med 1982; 306(4): 201-206.

3. Rowlison-Busza G and Epenetos AA. Citotoxicity following specific activation of amygdalin in monoclonal antibodies. Applications Clin Oncol 1992;179-183.

4. Syrigos KN, Rowlinson-Busza G and Epenetos AA. In vitro cytotoxicity following specific activation of amygdalin by beta-glucosidase conjugated to a bladder cancer-associated monoclonal antibody. Int J Cancer 1998;9;78(6):712-9.

5. Kousparou CA, Epenetos AA and Deonarain MP. Antibody-guided enzyme therapy of cancer producing cyanide results in necrosis of targeted cells. Int J Cancer 2002 May 1;99(1):138-48.

6. Inderst R. Systemic enzyme therapy. J Pharm 1992; 52.

7. Klein G, and Kullich W. Reducing pain by oral enzyme therapy in rheumatic diseases. Wien Med Wochenschr 1999;149(21-22):577-580.

Rakhimov MR. Anti-inflammatory activity of domestic papain. Eksp Klin Farmakol 2001;64(4);48-49.

Maurer HR. Bromelain:biochemistry, pharmacology and medical use. Cell Mol Life Sci 2001;58(9);1234-1245.

Emele JF et al. The analgesic-anti-inflammatory activity of papain. Arch Int Pharmacyn Ther 1966;159:126.

8. Maurer HR. Bromelain:biochemistry, pharmacology and medical use. Cell Mol Life Sci 2001;58(9);1234-1245.

Popiela T, Kulig J, Hanish J and Bock PR. Influence of a complementary treatment with oral enzymes on patients with colorectal cancer, an epidemiological retrolective cohort study. Cancer Chemother Pharmacol 2001;47(Suppl):S55-S63.

Beuth J, Ost B, Pakdaman A et al. Impact of complementary oral enzyme application on the postoperative treatment results of breast cancer patients results of an epidemiological multicentre retrolective cohort study. Cancer Chemother Pharmacol 2001;47(Suppl):S45-S54.

9. Popiela T, Kulig J, Hanish J and Bock PR. Influence of a complementary treatment with oral enzymes on patients with colorectal cancer, an epidemiological retrolective cohort study. Cancer Chemother Pharmacol 2001;47(Suppl):S55-S63.

Beuth J, Ost B, Pakdaman A et al. Impact of complementary oral enzyme application on the postoperative treatment results of breast cancer patients results of an epidemiological multicentre retrolective cohort study. Cancer Chemother Pharmacol 2001;47(Suppl):S45-S54.

Sakalova A, Bock PR, Dedik L et al. Retrolective cohort study of an additive therapy with an oral enzyme preparation in patients with multiple myeloma. Cancer Chemother Pharmacol 2001;47 (Suppl):S38-S44.

10. Maurer HR. Bromelain:biochemistry, pharmacology and medical use. Cell Mol Life Sci 2001;58(9);1234-1245.

Hale LP, Greer PK and Sempowski GD. Bromelain treatment alters leukocyte expression of cell surface molecules involved in cellular adhesion and activation. Clin Immunol 2002;104(2):183-190. Leipner J, and Saller R. Systemic enzyme therapy in oncology: effect and mode of action. Drugs 2000;59(4):769-780.

11. Maurer HR. Bromelain:biochemistry, pharmacology and medical use. Cell Mol Life Sci 2001;58(9);1234-1245.

12. Maurer HR. Bromelain:biochemistry, pharmacology and medical use. Cell Mol Life Sci 2001;58(9);1234-1245. Leipner J and Saller R. Systemic enzyme therapy in oncology: effect and mode of action. Drugs 2000;59(4):769-780.

13. Maurer HR. Bromelain:biochemistry, pharmacology and medical use. Cell Mol Life Sci 2001;58(9);1234-1245. Hiss WF. Enzymes in sport medicine and traumatology. J Natural Ther Methods (Zeitschrift für Naturheilmethoden) 1979: 2:1. Isaaksson JI and Ihse I: Pain reduction by oral pancreatic enzyme preparation in chronic pancreatitis. Dig Dis Sci 1983;28:97-102. Ransberger K. Enzyme treatment of immune complex disease. Arthritis and Rheumatism 1986; 8:16-19.

14. Steffen C and Menzel J. Enzyme consumption from immune complexes. J Rheumat (Zeitschrift fur Rheumatologie) 1989; 42;249-255.

15. Klein G et al. Clinical experience with enzyme therapy with rheumatoid arthritis in comparison with gold. Gen Med (Allgemeinmedizin) 1990; 19 (4): 144-147. Steffen C et al. Enzyme treatment in comparison with immune complex determinations in rheumatoid arthritis. Zeitschrift für Rheumatologie 1985;44:51-56. Neuhofer Ch. Enzyme therapy in multiple sclerosis. Hufeland J 1986;2:47-50.

16. Lane IW and Contreras E. High rate of bioactivity (reduction in gross tumor size) observed in advanced cancer patients treated with shark cartilage material. J of Naturopathic Med 1992;3:86-88.

17. Prudden JF et al. The acceleration of healing. Surg Gyn Obst 1969;128:1321-1326.

18. Feyzi R, Hassan ZM, Mostafai A. Modulation of CD (4)(+) and CD (8)(+) tumor infiltrating lymphocytes by a fraction isolated from shark cartilage: Shark cartilage modulates anti-tumor immunity. Int Inmunopharmacol 2003;3(7):921

19. Brem H and Folkman J. Inhibition of tumor angiogenesis mediated

by cartilage. J Exp Med 1975;141:427-439.

Davis PF et al. Inhibition of angiogenesis by oral ingestion of powdered shark cartilage in a rat model. Microvas Res 1997;54:178-182.

Folkman, J. Tumor angiogenesis: therapeutic implications. N Eng J Med 1971;285:1182-1186.

Lee A and Langer R. Shark cartilage contains inhibitors of tumor angiogenesis. Science. 1983;221:1185-1187.

20. Folkman, J. Tumor angiogenesis: therapeutic implications. N Eng J Med 1971;285:1182-1186.

21. Lee A and Langer R. Shark cartilage contains inhibitors of tumor angiogenesis. Science. 1983; 221:1185-1187.

22. Davis PF et al. Inhibition of angiogenesis by oral ingestion of powdered shark cartilage in a rat model. Microvas Res 1997;54:178-182.

Morris GM et al. Boron neutron capture of the rat 9L gliosarcoma: evaluation of the effects of shark cartilage. Br J Radial 2000;73:429-434.

23. Morris GM et al. Boron neutron capture of the rat 9L gliosarcoma: evaluation of the effects of shark cartilage. Br J Radial 2000; 73:429-434.

24. Barber R, Delahunt B, Grebe SK et al. Oral shark cartilage does not abolish carcinogenesis but delays progression in a murine model. Anticancer Res 2001;21(2A):1065-1069.

25. Dupont E et al. Angiostatic and antitumoral activity of NeovastatR, a molecular fraction derived from shark cartilage. Proc. Eighty-eight Annual Meeting. American Association of Cancer Research 1997;38 (Abstr 1530):226.

26. Ibid.

27. Mathews J. Media feeds frenzy over shark cartilage as cancer treatment. J Natl Cancer Inst 1993;85:1190-1191.

*Chapter 10 Something In The Air*

1. Pryor WA, Squadrito GL and Friedman M. The cascade mechanisms to explain ozone toxicity: The role of lipid ozonation products. Free Rad Biol Med 1995,19:935-941.

Bocci V. Does ozone therapy normalize the cellular redox balance?: Implications for the therapy of human immunodeficiency virus infection and several other diseases. Medical Hypotheses 1996,46:150-154.

2. Wells KH, Latino J, Gavalchin J and Poiesz B. Inactivation of human immunodeificiency virus type 1 by ozone in vitro. Blood 1991,78:1882-1890.

3. Bocci V. Does ozone therapy normalize the cellular redox balance?: Implications for the therapy of human immunodeficiency virus infection and several other diseases. Medical Hypotheses 1996,46:150-154.

4. Bocci V. Ozonization of blood for the therapy of viral disease and immunodeficiencies. A hypothesis. Medical Hypotheses 1992,39:30-34.

5. Bocci V. Is ozone therapy therapeutic? Perspectives in Biology and Medicine 1998,42:131-143.

6. Wells KH, Latino J, Gavalchin J and Poiesz B. Inactivation of human immunodeificiency virus type 1 by ozone in vitro. Blood 1991,78:1882-1890.
   Carpendale TF, and Freeberg JK. Ozone inactivates HIV at noncytotoxic concentrations. Antiviral Res 1991,16:281-292.

7. Bocci V. Does ozone therapy normalize the cellular redox balance?: Implications for the therapy of human immunodeficiency virus infection and several other diseases. Medical Hypotheses 1996,46:150-154.
   Hernández F, Menéndez S and Wong R. Decrease of blood cholesterol and stimulation of antioxidative response in cardiophathy patients treated with endovenous ozone therapy. Free Rad Biol Med 1995,19(1):115-119.

8. Di Paolo N, Bocci V, Garosi G et al. Extracorporeal blood oxygenation and ozonation (EBOO) in man. Preliminary report. Int J Artif Organs 2000; 23(2):131-141.

9. Coppola L, Verrazzo G, Giunta R et al. Oxygen/ozone therapy and haemorheological parameters in peripheral chronic arterial occlusive disease. Throm Arterioscler 1992,8:83-90.
   Tylicki L, Nieweglowski T, Biedunkiewicz B et al. Beneficial clinical effects of ozonated autohemotherapy in chronically dialysed patients with atherosclerotic ischemia of the lower limbs-pilot study. Int J Artif Organs 2001; 24:79-82.
   Hernández F, Menéndez S and Wong R. Decrease of blood cholesterol and stimulation of antioxidative response in cardiophathy patients treated with endovenous ozone therapy. Free Rad Biol Med 1995; 19(1):115-119.

Di Paolo N, Bocci V, Garosi G et al. Extracorporeal blood oxygenation and ozonation (EBOO) in man. Preliminary report. Int J Artif Organs 2000; 23(2):131-141.

10. Pryor WA, Squadrito GL and Friedman M. The cascade mechanisms to explain ozone toxicity: The role of lipid ozonation products. Free Rad Biol Med 1995,19:935-941.

Pryor WA. Mechanisms of radical formation from reactions of ozone with target molecules in the lung. Free Rad Biol Med 1994, 17:451-465.

11. See note 5.

12. Bocci V. Is ozone therapy therapeutic? Perspectives in Biology and Medicine 1998,42:131-143.

Di Paolo N, Bocci V, Garosi G et al. Extracorporeal blood oxygenation and ozonation (EBOO) in man. Preliminary report. Int J Artif Organs 2000,23(2):131-141.

Bocci V, Valacchi G, Corradeschi F et al. Studies on the biological effects of ozone; 7. Generation of reactive oxygen species (ROS) after exposure of human blood to ozone. J Biol Reg Homeost Agents 1998, 12(3):67-75.

13. *Nitric oxide:* A gas molecule that is critical to numerous biological processes, including vasodilaton, neurotransmission and tumor-killing.

14. Bocci V. Is ozone therapy therapeutic? Perspectives in Biology and Medicine 1998,42:131-143.

Bocci V, Luzzi E, Corradeshi F et al. Studies on the biological effects of ozone: 3. An attempt to define conditions for optimal induction of cytokines. Lymphokine and Cytokine Research 1993, 12 (2):121-126.

Bocci V, Valacchi G, Corradeschi F and Fanetti G. Studies on the biological effects of ozone: 8. Effects on the total antioxidant status and on interleukin-8 production. Mediators of Inflammation 1998; 7:313-317.

Bocci V and Paulesu L. Studies on the biological effects of ozone: 1. Induction of interferon gamma on human leucocytes. Haematologica 1990, 75:510-515.

Paulesu L, Luzzi E and Bocci V. Studies on the biological effects of ozone: 2. Induction of tumor necrosis factor (TNF) on human leucocytes. Lymphokyne and Cytokine Research 1991; 10:409-412.

Valacchi and Bocci V. Studies on the biological effects of ozone: 11. Releasing factors from human endothelial cells. Mediators of Inflammation 2000; 9 (6): 271-276.

15. See note 4.

16. Toyokuni S, Okamoto K, Yodoi J and Hiai H. Persistent oxidative stress in cancer. FEBS Letters 1995, 358: 1-3.

Ames BN, Shigenaga MK and Hagen TM. Oxidants, antioxidants, and the degenerative diseases of aging. Proc Nat Acad Sci USA 1993; 90:7915-7922.

Schwarz KB. Oxidative stress during viral infection: A review. Free Rad Biol Mcd 1996; 21:641-649.

Simonian NA and Coyle JT. Oxidative stress in neurodegenerative diseases. Ann Rev Pharmacol Toxicol 1996; 36:83-106.

*Chapter 11 Seeing The Light*

1. Laurens H. The Physiologic effects of ultraviolet irradiation. JAMA 1938; 11:2390-2391.

2. Knott EK. Development of ultraviolet blood irradiation. Am J Surg 1948, LXXVI: 165-171.

3. Barger G, and Knott EK. Blood: Ultraviolet irradiation (Knott technic). Med Physics 1950, 11:132-136.

4. Fratantoni J and Prodouz K. Viral inactivation of blood products. Transfusion 1990;30(6): 480-481.

5. Corash L and Hanson C. Guest Editorial. Photoinactivation of viruses and cells for medical applications. Blood Cells 1992;18:3-5.

6. Frick G and Linke A. Ultraviolet irradiation of the blood, its development and current status. Z Arztl Fortbild 1986;80(11);441-444.

7. Marochkov AV, Doronin VA and Kravtsov NN. Complications in ultraviolet irradiation of the blood. Anesteziol Reanimatol 1990;4:55-56.

8. Edelson RL et al. Treatment of leukemic cutaneous T-cell lymphoma with extracorporeally- photoactivated 8-methoxypsoralen. N Eng J Med 1987;316:297-303.

9. Bisaccia E et al. Extracorporeal photochemotherapy alone or with adjuvant therapy in the treatment of cutaneous T-cell lymphoma. A 9-year retrospective study at a single institution. J Am Acad Dermatol 2000;43:263-271.

Duvic M et al. Photopheresis therapy for cutaneous T-cell lymphoma. J Am Acad Dermatol 1996; 35:573-579.

Zic J et al. Long-term follow-up with cutaneous T-cell lymphoma. J Am Acad Dermatol 1996;35;935-945.

10. Barr ML, Meiser B, et al. Photopheresis for the prevention or rejection in cardiac transplantation. N Eng J Med 1998;339:1744-1751. Knobler RM, Graninger W et al. Extracorporeal photochemotherapy for the treatment of systemic lupus erythematosus a pilot study. Arthritis Rheum 1992; 35:319-323.

11. Song PS and Tapley KJ. Photochemistry and photobiology of psoralens. Photchem Photobiol 1979;29:1177-1197.

12. Song PS and Tapley KJ. Photochemistry and photobiology of psoralens. Photchem Photobiol 1979;29:1177-1197. Edelson Rl. Editorial. Transimmunization: the science catches up to the clinical success. Transfus Apheresis Sci 2002;26:177-180.

13. Edelson Rl. Editorial. Transimmunization: the science catches up to the clinical success. Transfus Apheresis Sci 2002;26:177-180.

14. Timmerman JM, and Levy R. Dendritic cell vaccines for cancer immunotherapy. Annu Rev Med 1999,50:507-529.

15. Ibid.

16. Yoshiki T, Naohiro S et al. Photoactivational cytokine-modulatory action of 8-methoxypsoralen plus ultraviolet A in lymphocytes, monocytes, and cutaneous T cells lymphoma cells. Ann NY Acad Sci 2001;941:185-193.

17. Berger CL, Xu A-L et al. Induction of human tumor-loaded dendritic cells. Int J Cancer 2001:91:438-447.

18. Burdin N and Moingeon P. Cancer vacines based on dendritic cells loaded with tumor-associated antigens. Cell Biol Toxicol 2001;17(2):67-75. Whitside TL and Odoux C. Dendritic cell biology and cancer therapy. Cancer Immunol Immunother 2004;53(3):240-248. Tsan MF and Gao B. Cytokine function of heat shock proteins. Am J Physiol Cell Physiol 2004;286(4):C739-744. Kantengwa S, Jornot L, Devenoges C and Nicod LP. Superoxide anions induce the maturation of human dendritic cells. Am J Respir Crit Care Med 2003;167(3):431-437. Rutault K, Alderman C, Chain BM and Katz DR. Reactive oxygen species activate human peripheral blood dendritic cells. Free Radic Bio Med 1999;26(1-2):232-238. Leon B, Martinez Del Hoyo G, Parrillas V et al. Dendritic cell differ-

entiation potential of mouse monocytes: monocytes represent immediate precursors of CD8- and CD8+ splenic dendritic cells. Blood 2004;103: 2668-2676.

Albert ML, Sauter B and Bhardwaj N. Dendritic cells acquire antigen from apoptotic cells and induce class 1-restricted CTLs. Nature 1998;392(6671):86-89.

19. Yoo EK, Rook AH et al. Apoptosis induction by ultraviolet A and photochemotherapy in cutaneous T-cell lymphoma. Relevance in mechanism of therapeutic action. J Invest Dermatol 1996;107:235-242.

20. Berger CL, Xu A-L et al. Induction of human tumor-loaded dendritic cells. Int J Cancer 2001:91:438-447.

21. Berger CL, Hanlon D et al. Transimmunization, a novel approach for tumor immunotherapy. Transfus Apheresis Sci 2002;26:205-216. Girardi M, Schechner J et al. Transimmunization and the evolution of extracorporeal photochemotherapy. Transfus Apheresis Sci 2002;26;181-190.

*Chapter 13 Mind Medicine*

1. See Dr. Ernesto Contreras' autobiography, *To you, my beloved patient.* (Chula Vista, CA Interpacific Press) 1999.

2. http://www.musicasmedicine.com/aboutmt.htm

3. Cousins, Norman. *Anatomy of an Illness. As perceived by the patient.* (New York:Bantam Books) 1989 [1979].

4. Deane K, Fitch M and Carman M. An innovative art therapy program for cancer patients. Can Oncol Nurs J. 2000 Fall;10(4):147-51, 152-7.

5. Ishihara S, Makita S, Imai M, Hashimoto, T and Nohara R. Relationship between natural killer activity and anger expression in patients with coronary heart disease. Heart Vessels 2003;18(2), 85-92.

6. Study: depression, sadness weaken immune system. February 17, 2004 http://www.thedenverchannel.com/print/2448536/detail.html

7. Bennett MP, Zeller JM, Rosenberg L and McCann J. The effect of mirthful laughter on stress and natural killer cell activity. Alternative Therapy Health Medicine 2003; 9(2), 38-45.

8. Mayr B and Mayr A. Interactions between the immune system and the psyche. Tierarztl Prax Ausg K Klientiere Heimtiere 1998;26(4), 230-235.

9. See note 6.
10. Frankl V. *Man's search for meaning*. (Boston, MA: Beacon Press) 1959.

*Chapter 15 True Spirit*

1. See Byrd RC.Positive therapeutic effects of intercessory prayer in a coronary care unit population. South Med J. 1988 Jul;81(7):826-9.

   Tatsumura Y, Maskarinec G, Shumay DM and Kakai H. Religious and spiritual resources, CAM, and conventional treatment in the lives of cancer patients. Altern Ther Health Med 2003 May-Jun;9(3):64-71.

   Kennedy JE, Abbott RA and Rosenberg BS. Changes in spirituality and well-being in a retreat program for cardiac patients: Altern Ther Health Med 2002;8(4):64-6, 68-70, 72-73.

   OG Harding . The healing power of intercessory prayer.West Indian Med J; 2001; 50(4): 269-72.

   JA Astin, E Harkness and E Ernst .The efficacy of "distant healing": a systematic review of randomized trials. Ann Intern Med 2000; 132(11): 903-10.

*Appendices*

1. Fukuda T, Ito H, Mukainaka T et al. Anti-tumor promoting effect of glycosides from Prunus persica seed. Biol Pharm Bull 2003;26(2):271-273.

   Egli KL. Colorimetric determination of cyanide liberated from apricot kernels. J Assoc Off Anal Chem 1977;60 (4):954-956.

   Frakes RA, Sharma RP and Willhite CC. Comparative metabolism of linamarin and amygalin in hamsters. Food Chem Toxicol 1986;24(5):417-420.

2. Malgorzata Iciek and Lidia Wlodek. Biosynthesis and biological properties of compounds containing highly reactive, reduced sulfuna sulfur. Pol J Pharmacol 2001;53:215-255.

3. Nagahara N, Ito T and Minami M. Mercaptopyruvate sulfurtransferase as a defense against cyanide intoxication: molecular properties and mode of detoxification. Histol Histopathol 1999;14(4):1277-1286.

   Porter DW, Nealley EW and Baskin SI. In vivo detoxification of cyanide by cistathionase gamma-lyase. Biochem Pharmacol 1996;52(6):941-944.

4. Spallarossa A, Forlani F, Carpen A et al. The "rhodanese" fold and

catalytic mechanism of 3-mercaptopyruvate sulfurtranferases:crystal structure of SseA from Escherichia coli. J Mol Biol 2004; 335(2):583-593.

Nagahara N, Okazaki T and Nishino T. Cytosolic mercaptopyruvate sulfurtransferase is evolutionarily related to mitochondrial rhodanese. Striking similarity in active site amino acid sequence and the increase in the mercaptopyruvate sulfurtranferase activity of rhodanese by site-directed mutagenesi. J Biol Chem 1995;270(27):16230-16235.

Bordo D, Bork P. The rhodanese/Cdc25 phosphatase superfamily. Sequence-structure-function relations. EMBO Rep 2002;3(8):741-746.

5. Wrobel M, Ubuka T, Yao WB and Abe T. Effects of thyroxine on L-cysteine desulfuratuon in mouse liver. Acta Med Okayama 2000;54(1):9-14.

6. Smith PF, Booker BM, Creaven P et al. Pharmacokinetics and pharmacodynamics of mesna-mediated plasma cystcine depletion. J Clin Pharmacol 2003;43(12):1324-1328.

Lauterburg BH, Nguyen T, Hartmann B et al. Depletion of total cysteine, glutathione, and homocysteine in plasma by ifosfamide/mesna therapy. Cancer Chemother Pharmacol 1994;35(2):132-136.

Stofer-Vogel B, Cerny T, Kupfer A et al. Depletion of circulating cyst(e)ine by oral and intravenous mesna. Br J Cancer 1993;68(3):590-593.

Komlosh A, Volohonsky G, Porat N et al. Gamma-glutamyl transpeptidase and glutathione biosynthesis in non-tumoregenic and tumoregenic rat liver oval cell lines. Carcinogenesis 2001;22(12):2009-2016.

Miller LT, Watson WH, Kirlin WG et al. Oxidation of the glutathione/glutathione disulfide redox state is induced by cysteine deficiency in human colon carcinoma HT29 cells. J Nutr 2002;132(8):2303-2306.

Deplancke B and Gaskins HR. Redox control of the transsulfuration and glutathione biosynthesis pathways. Curr Opin Clin Nutr Metab Care 2002;5(1):85-92.

Ahmad S, Okine L, Wood R et al. gamma-Glutamyl traspeptidase (gamma-GT) and maintenance of thiol pools in tumor cells resistant to alkylating agents. J Cell Physiol 1987;131(2):240-246.

7. Miller LT, Watson WH, Kirlin WG et al. Oxidation of the glutathione/glutathione disulfide redox state is induced by cysteine deficiency in

human colon carcinoma HT29 cells. J Nutr 2002;132(8):2303-2306.

Carretero J, Obrador E, Anasagasti MJ et al. Growth-associated changes in glutathione content correlate with liver metastatic activity of B16 melanoma cells. Clin Exp Metastasis 1999;17(7):567-574.

Wu G, Fang YS, Yang S et al. Glutathione metabolism and its implication for health. J Nutr 2004;134(3):489-492.

Griffith OW. Biologic and pharmacologic regulation of mammalian glutathione synthesis. Free Radic Biol Med 1999;27(9-10):922-935.

8. Zhang JG, Tirmenstein MA, Nicholl-Grzemski FA and Fariss MW. Mitochondrial electron transport inhibitors cause lipid peroxidation-dependent and –indepent cell death: protective role of antioxidants. Arch Biochem Biophys 2001;393(1):87-96.

Armstrong JS, Steinauer KK, Hornug B et al. Role of glutathione depletion and reactive oxygen species generation in apoptotic signaling in a human B lymphoma cell line. Cell Death Differ 2002;9(3);252-263.

Swamy SM and Huat BT. Intracellular glutathione depletion and reactive oxygen species generation are important in apha-hederin-induced apoptosis of P388 cells. Mol Cell Biochem 2003;245(1-2):127-139.

Macho A, Hirsch T, Marzo I et al. Glutathione depletion is an early and calcium elevation is a late event of thymocyte apoptosis. J Immunol 1997;158(10):4612-4619.

Fleury C, Mignotte B and Vayssiere JL. Mitochondrial reactive oxygen species in cell death signaling. Biochimie 2002;84(2-3):131-141.

Merad-Boudia M, Nicole A, Santiard-Baron D et al. Mitochondrial impairment as an early event in the process of apoptosis induced by glutathione depletion in neuronal cells: relevance to Parkinson's disease. Biochem Pharmacol 1998;56(5):645-655.

Wullner U, Seyfried J, Groscurth P et al. Glutathione depletion and neuronal cell death: the role of reactive oxygen intermediates and mitochondrial function. Brain Res 1999;826(1):53-62

9. Ida T, Kijima H, Urata Y et al. Hammerhead ribozyme against gamma-glutamylcysteine synthetase sensitizes human colonic cancer cells to cisplatin by down regulating both the glutathione synthesis and the expression of multidrug resistance proteins. Cancer Gene Ther

2001;8(10):803-814.

Kigawa J, Minagawa Y, Cheng X and Terakawa N. Gamma-glutamyl cysteine synthetase up-regulates glutahione and multidrug resistance-associated protein in patients with chemoresitant epithelial ovarian cancer. Clin Cancer Res 1998;4(7):1737-1741.

Homolya L, Varadi A and Sarkadi B. Multidrug resistance-associated proteins. Export pumps for conjugates with glutathione, glucoronate or sulfate. Biofactors 2003;17(1-4):103-114.

Rappa G, Gamesik MP, Mitina Rl et al. Retroviral transfer of MRP1 and gamma-glutamyl cysteine synthetase, modulates cell sensitivity to L-buthionine-S,R-sulphoximine (BSO): new rationale for the use of BSO in cancer therapy. Eur J Cancer 2003;39(1):120-128.

Calvert P, Yao KS, Hamilton TC and OD'wyer PJ. Clinical studies of reversal of drug resistance based on glutathione. Chem Biol Interact 1998;111-112:213-224.

Rudin CM, Yang Z, Schumaker LM et al. Inhibition of glutathione synthesis reverses Bcl-2-mediated cisplatin resistance. Cancer Res 2003;63(2):312-318.

Hatcher EL, Chen Y and Kang YJ. Cadmium resistance in A549 cells correlates with elevated glutathione content but not antioxidant enzymatic activities. Free Radic Biol Med 1995;19(6):805-812.

el-akawi Z, Abu-hadid M, Perez R et al. Altered glutathione metabolism in oxaliplatin resistant ovarian carcinoma cells. Cancer Lett 1996;105(1):5-14.

Britten RA, Green JA and Warenius HM. Cellular glutathione (GSH) and glutathione S-tranferase (GST) activity in human ovarian tumor biopsies following exposure to alkylating agents. Int J Radiat Oncol Biol Phys 1992;24(3):527-531.

10. Smith PF, Booker BM, Creaven P et al. Pharmacokinetics and pharmacodynamics of mesna-mediated plasma cysteine depletion. J Clin Pharmacol 2003;43(12):1324-1328.

Kabaskal L, Ozker K, Hayward M et al. Technetium-99m sestamibi uptake in human breast carcinoma cell lines displaying glutathione-associated drug-resistance. Eur J Nucl Med 1996;23(5):568-570.

Perek N, Koumanov F, Denoyer D et al. Modulation of the multidrug resistance of glioma by glutahione levels depletion—interaction with Tc-99M-Sestamibi and Tc-99M-Tetrofosmin. Cancer Biother Radiopharm 2002;17(3):291-302.

Denoyer D, Perek N, Le Jeune N et al. The multidrug resistance of in vitro tumor cell lines derived from human breast carcionama MCF-7 does not influence pentavalent technetium-99m-dimercaptosuccinic Acid uptake. Cancer Biother Radiopharm 2003;1885):791-801.

Anasagasti MJ, Martin JJ, Mendoza L et al. Glutathione protects metastatic melanoma cells against oxidative stress in the murine hepatic microvasculature. Hepatology 1998;27(5):1249-1256.

11. Pendyala L, Schwartz G, Smith P et al. Modulation of plasma thiols and mixed disulfides by BNP7787 in patients receiving paclitaxel/cisplatin therapy. Cancer Chemother Pharmacol 2003;51(5):376-384.

Hoffman A, Spetner LM and Burke M. Redox-regulated mechanism may account for zerumbones' ability to suppress cancer-cell proliferatuon. Carcinogeneis 2002;23(5):795-802.

Sugiyama T and Sadzuka Y. Theanine and glutamate transporter inhibitor enhance the antitumor efficacy of chemotherapeutic agents. Biochem Biophys Acta 2003;1653(2):47-59.

Palomares T, Bilbao P, del Olmo M et al. In vitro and in vivo comparison between the effects of treatment with adenosine triphosphate and treatment with buthionine sulfoximine on chemosensitization and tumor growth of B16 melanoma. Melanoma Res 1999;9(3):233-242.

Revesz L, Edgren MR and Wainson AA. Selective toxicity of buthionine sulfoximine (BSO) to melanoma cells in vitro and in vivo. Int J Radiat Oncol Biol Phys 1994; 29(2):403-406.

Sen CK. Redox signaling and the emerging therapeutic potential of thiol antioxidants. Biochem Pharmacol 1998;55(11):1747-1758.

12. Kang JS, Cho D, Kim YI et al. L-ascorbic acid (vitamin C) induces the apoptosis of B16 murine melanoma cells via a caspase-8-independent pathway. Cancer Immunol Immunother 2003;52(11):693-698.

Gao F, Yi J, Shi G et al. Ascorbic acid enhances the apoptosis of U937 cell induced by arsenic trioxide in combination with DMNQ and its mechanism Zhonghua Xue Ye Xue Za Zhi 2002;23(1):9-11.

Grad JM, Bahlis NJ and Boise LH. Ascorbic acid augments arsenic-mediated cell death in multiple myeloma (mm) cells. Scientific WorldJournal 2001; 1(1 Suppl 3):110.

Bahlis NJ, McCafferty-Grad J, Jordan-McMurry I et al. Feasibility and correlates of arsenic trioxide combined with ascorbic acid-mediated depletion of intracellular glutathione for the treatment of relapsed/refractory multiple myeloma. Clin Cancer Res 2002;8(12):3643-3645.

Grad JM, Bahlis NJ, Reis L et al. Ascorbic acid enhances arsenic trioxide-induced cytotoxicity in multiple myeloma cells. Blood 2001;98(3):805-813.

Lasalvia-Prisco E, Cucchi S, Vazquez J et al. Serum markers variation consistent with autoschizis induced by ascorbic acid-medianone in patients with prostate cancer. Med Oncol 2003;20(1):45-52.

De Loecker W, Janssens J, Bonte J and Taper HS. Effects of sodium ascorbate (vitamin C) and 2-methyl-1,4-naphtoquinone (vitamin K3) treatment on human tumor cell growth in vitro. II. Synergism with combined chemotherapy action. Anticancer Res 1993;13(1):103-106.

Gilloteaux J, Jamison JM, Venugopal M et al. Scanning electron microscopy and transmission electron microscopy aspects of synergistic antitumor activity of vitamin C, vitamin K3 combinations against human prostatic carcinoma cells. Scanning Micros 1995;9(1):159-173.

Calderon PB, Cadrobbi J, Marquez C et al. Potential therapeutic application of the association of vitamin C and K3 in cancer treatment. Curr Med Chem 2002;9(24):2271-2285.

Verrax J, Cadrobbi J, Delvaux M et al. The association of vitamins C and K3 kills cancer cells mainly by autoschizis, a novel form of cell death. Basis for their potential use as coadjuvants in anticancer therapy. Eur J Med Chem 2003;38(5):451-457.

May JM, Qu X and Li X. Requirement for GSH on recycling of ascorbic acid in endothelial cells. Biochem Pharmacol 2001;62(7):873-881.

May JM, Qu ZC, Neel DR and Li X. Recycling of vitamin C from its oxidized forms by human endothelial cells.

13. Auriga M and Koj A. Protective effect of rhodanese on the respiration of isolated mitochondria intoxicated with cyanide. Bull Polish Sci Ser Biol 1975; 23(5):305-310.

Himwich NH and Saunders JP. Enzymatic conversion of cyanide to thiocyanate. Am J Physiol 1948;153:348-354.

Krebs, Jr E. Laetrile's pioneer —a definitive statement on the theory and action of Vitamin B-17. The Choice 1977;3(6):12-14.

Krebs ET. The nitrilosides (Vitamin B-17), their nature, occurrence and metabolic significance anti-neoplastic Vitamin B-17. J Appl Nutr 1970;22:75-86.

Manner HW. The non-toxicity of Amygdalin to laboratory mice. Sci Biol J 1977; 347-349.

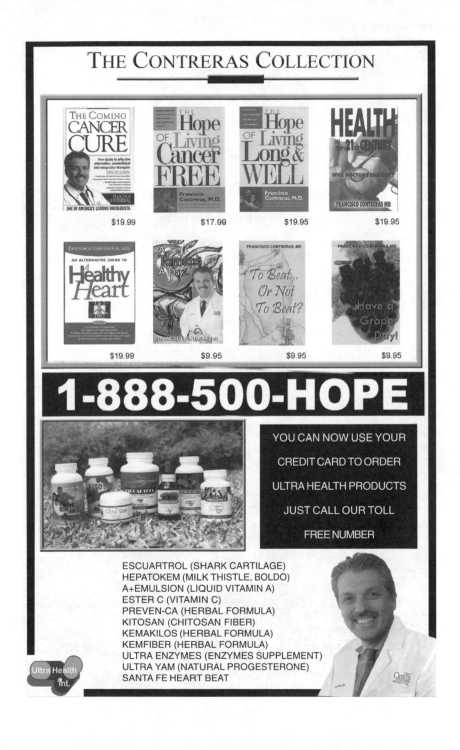

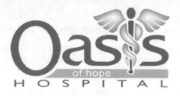

# DID YOU HAVE TO PAY FOR YOUR TREATMENT OUT OF YOUR OWN POCKET?

Insurance Claims Filing Services is a company that specializes in the filing of foreign health insurance claims.

A major concern all patients have is the extent to which their insurance companies will pay their medical services.

We have 15 years of experience in the insurance coordinating field, and have been over 90% successful in collecting on claims we file.

We look foward to assisting you. If you should have any questions, please call us at 713/937-1875. For immediate transmission of documents, please fax your information to 713/937-1921 or e-mail at claimsfiling@hotmail.com.

*Insurance Claims Filing Services*

*P.O. Box 91036-133*
*Houston, TX 77291-1036*
*713/937-1875*
*FAX 713/937-1921*
*claimsfiling@hotmail.com*

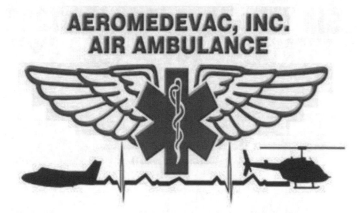

# Aeromedevac, Inc.

4420 Rainier Ave. Ste. 200

San Diego, Ca. 92120

*Toll free from the U.S.* 800. 462-0911

*Toll free from Mexico.* 001.800.832.5087

*Local:* 619.284.7910

*Fax:* 619.284.7918

## www.aeromedevac.com